EuropeActive's Essentials for Fitness Instructors

EuropeActive

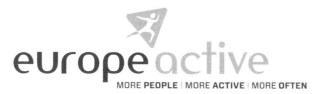

MORE **PEOPLE** | MORE **ACTIVE** | MORE **OFTEN**

Rita Santos Rocha
Alfonso Jiménez
Thomas Rieger

EDITORS

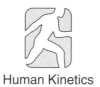

Human Kinetics

Library of Congress Cataloging-in-Publication Data

EuropeActive.

 EuropeActive's essentials for fitness instructors / EuropeActive ; Rita Sanchos Rocha, Thomas Rieger, Alfonso Jiménez, editors.

     pages cm

 Includes bibliographical references and index.

 1. Physical fitness--Handbooks, manuals, etc. 2. Physical fitness--Physiological aspects. 3. Exercise--Physiological aspects--Handbooks, manuals, etc. 4. Health--Handbooks, manuals, etc. 5. Physical education and training--European Union countries. I. Rocha, Rita Santos, 1971- II. Rieger, Thomas, 1973- III. Jiménez, Alfonso, 1970- IV. Title.

 GV481.E76 2015

 613.7094--dc23

                                    2014029350

ISBN: 978-1-4504-2379-3 (print)

The web addresses cited in this text were current as of November, 2014, unless otherwise noted.

Acquisitions Editor: Roger Earle; **Developmental Editor:** Kevin Matz; **Associate Managing Editor:** Nicole Moore; **Copyeditor:** Joy Wotherspoon; **Indexer:** Katy Balcer; **Permissions Manager:** Dalene Reeder; **Graphic Designers:** Nancy Rasmus and Dawn Sills; **Cover Designer:** Keith Blomberg; **Photographs (interior):** © Human Kinetics, unless otherwise noted; **Photo Asset Manager:** Laura Fitch; **Photo Production Manager:** Jason Allen; **Art Manager:** Kelly Hendren; **Associate Art Manager:** Alan L. Wilborn; **Illustrations:** © Human Kinetics, unless otherwise noted; **Printer:** Sheridan Books

Printed in the United States of America   10 9 8 7 6 5 4 3 2 1

The paper in this book is certified under a sustainable forestry program.

Human Kinetics
Website: www.HumanKinetics.com

United States: Human Kinetics
P.O. Box 5076
Champaign, IL 61825-5076
800-747-4457
e-mail: humank@hkusa.com

Canada: Human Kinetics
475 Devonshire Road Unit 100
Windsor, ON N8Y 2L5
800-465-7301 (in Canada only)
e-mail: info@hkcanada.com

Europe: Human Kinetics
107 Bradford Road
Stanningley
Leeds LS28 6AT, United Kingdom
+44 (0) 113 255 5665
e-mail: hk@hkeurope.com

Australia: Human Kinetics
57A Price Avenue
Lower Mitcham, South Australia 5062
08 8372 0999
e-mail: info@hkaustralia.com

New Zealand: Human Kinetics
P.O. Box 80
Torrens Park, South Australia 5062
0800 222 062
e-mail: info@hknewzealand.com

E5642

Contents

Preface

EuropeActive, located in Brussels, is the leading not-for-profit organisation representing the European health and fitness sector. EuropeActive is also a standards-setting body that promotes best practice in instruction and training with the ultimate objective to raise the quality of service and improve customers' exercise experience and results. This task is formally implemented by the Standards Council, the independent body of EuropeActive that provides strategic guidance in relation to standards for people, programmes and places. The main activity of the Standards Council in the past few years has been the development of the aforementioned standards in education and training to define the skills and knowledge required for people working in the fitness industry. It is part of the process of developing a sector framework, which in turn is based on the eight levels of the European Qualifications Framework (EQF).

The EQF links countries' qualifications systems together, acting as a translation device to make qualifications more understandable. This will help learners and workers wishing to move between countries, change jobs or move between educational institutions at home.

In addition, EuropeActive fully supports the strategic principles and objectives of the EU Lifelong Learning Programme. Currently, the sector qualifications framework contains the formally published standards for all vocational levels from 2 to 5 (visit www.ehfa.eu.com).

The education behind these standards should be grounded in EuropeActive's Code of Ethical Practice (included in *EuropeActive's Foundations for Exercise Professionals*), which describes the principles of ethical behaviour in exercise instruction, including rights, relationships, personal responsibilities and professional standards. Moreover, it informs and protects members of the public and customers using the services of exercise professionals.

The present book is the second in a series containing the following three titles:

EuropeActive's Foundations for Exercise Professionals
EuropeActive's Essentials for Fitness Instructors
EuropeActive's Essentials for Personal Trainers

The series reflects the current status of educational fitness standards in Europe and provides the foundations at EQF level 2, following with the essentials for fitness instructors at EQF level 3 and for personal trainers at EQF level 4. Hence, *EuropeActive's Essentials for Fitness Instructors* provides the educational competences for instructors at EQF level 3 and is based on *EuropeActive's Foundations for Exercise Professionals.*

Chapter 1 explains the importance of customer service in the saturated fitness market. Service-oriented instructors apply customers' expectations to the training process and monitor the results. Chapter 2 explains the importance of instructors' communication skills in influencing the quality of intervention in fitness training. Chapter 3 focuses on the cardiovascular responses to exercise. Fitness instructors must understand the basic physiological concepts and be able to apply each concept to clients' exercise programmes to ensure safety and effectiveness. Chapter 4 reviews the factors in analyzing human motion and minimizing risk of injury during resistance training. Also discussed are the general safety procedures and spotting techniques for effective resistance training, the importance of evaluating training status for designing appropriate resistance training programmes and assessing the rate of progression and adaptation. Chapter 5 approaches exercise prescription based on ability and explains the changes that take place after the progressive exercise. The principles of training are also addressed. Chapter 6 describes the basic requirements that instructors should consider before starting an exercise programme in order to ensure effectiveness and safety. Chapter 7 describes the principles of conducting the group fitness workouts and explains why the instructor must present exercises with enthusiasm. Chapter 8 presents the characteristics of effective use of music in a fitness class. Music guides the instructor and motivates participants, so choosing appropriate music is vital. Chapter 9 further explores the use of music based on intensity and fitness goals and the planning of appropriate choreography. Chapter 10 prepares instructors to end sessions properly. The end of class is not just the mere conclusion to exercise training associated with cooling down and stretching. It is the perfect opportunity to invite clients to a follow-up class. Chapter 11 describes the basic requirements of programming the class that the instructor should consider before starting a group fitness class. Chapter 12 identifies and describes several relaxation techniques that can be used for stress management.

This book was developed and written by EuropeActive's Standards Council in coordination with many renowned experts in exercise and sport science worldwide. Thus, the content mirrors the current state of research as well as the actual requirements of the European fitness sector.

The Standards Council of EuropeActive sincerely thank all those involved in this project, especially editors and authors, for their willingness to contribute.

Rita Santos Rocha, second vice chair
EuropeActive Standards Council

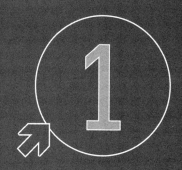

Customer Service

Thomas Rieger

Fitness centres all over Europe provide high-quality services to promote health and well-being. The industry also has economic significance. Despite the increasing number of customers, growing industry revenue, and number of providers, many providers face a central problem: high customer fluctuation (German Fitness Gym Association 2013; Rieger 2009, 2011). Specifically, customers may cancel their membership, change providers, or skip sporting activity completely. As a result, it is becoming increasingly difficult for fitness centres to retain customers.

What reasons account for this problem? Research shows a positive relationship between the level of satisfaction experienced by customers and their loyalty to a provider (Alexandris et al. 2004; Bodet 2008; Hallowell 1996; Homburg and Koschate 2007; Zeithaml et al. 2012). Many other studies emphasise that customer satisfaction depends strongly on the quality of customer service (Anderson et al. 1994; Grönroos 2007; Schneider and Bowen 1995); furthermore, different studies show comparable results concerning customer service in the fitness centre industry (Afthinos et al. 2005; Howat et al. 1996; Lagrosen and Lagrosen 2007; Moxham and Wiseman 2009; Tsitskari et al. 2006). Thus, providers in the saturated fitness market need to master customer service concepts that allow them to fulfil customers' expectations.

Principles of Customer Service

According to Grönroos (2007), a service is 'an activity or series of activities of more or less intangible nature that normally, but not necessarily, take place in interactions between the customers and service employees and/or physical resources or goods and/or systems of the service provider, which are provided as solutions to customer problems' (p. 52). Meffert and Bruhn (2008) take an even more comprehensive approach that includes an outcome category (see figure 1.1).

In Meffert and Bruhn's (2008) model, services are formulated in terms of three phases:

1. Potential orientation (internal factors, such as facilities, equipment or qualification of employees)
2. Process orientation (combination of internal and external factors in the delivery process)
3. Outcome orientation (effects of the delivery process, e.g., satisfaction)

Customers pay for services in order to address or solve their problems. Therefore, providers must obtain information about their customers' needs in order to deliver high-quality service. With this focus, providers must pay attention to tangible factors involved in their service, like facilities or equipment.

The importance of potential orientation steps into the foreground when the presence of the customer is essential for the service delivery, as with fitness sports. The customer's perceptions of the intangible delivery process can be influenced by the previously mentioned tangible features (Bitner 1992). For example, a state-of-the-art facility with up-to-date workout equipment could give potential customers positive associations with the provided services. Important details to consider include the equipment and the interior design of rooms and other areas like the locker room or spa centre. Comfort and beauty

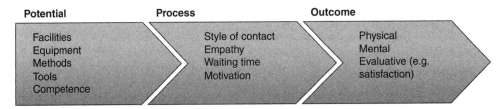

Figure 1.1   Phases of fitness services.
Adapted from Meffert and Bruhn 2008.

create positive impressions in a service environment. The phase of process orientation illuminates the concrete interaction between the instructor and customer, and success hinges on the human performance of instructors in this situation (Grönroos 2007; Zeithaml et al. 2008). It is based on the typical characteristics of the service as a product: simultaneously producing and consuming a heterogeneous performance from the provider (e.g., know-how, physical capability), integration of external factors and immateriality (Meffert and Bruhn 2008; Zeithaml et al. 2008). The behaviour, attitude and interpersonal skills of the instructor are of vital importance. Besides having good communication skills, instructors should be friendly, obliging and customer oriented. All of these soft features can affect interaction with customers and influence the service outcome (Lengnick-Hall 1996; Rieger 2011). The process is the primary objective of a fitness service. The instructor must be aware of the importance of interpersonal connections. Expertise alone is not enough. The instructor needs a fundamental knowledge of human nature in order to be empathetic. Friendliness and courtesy are a must.

Instructors must intensively manage the core element of the so-called 'human–human interface' (Ko and Pastore 2004). The close and almost intimate relationship with customers requires instructors to cultivate empathy and a comprehensive knowledge of human nature. If an exercise customer wants to achieve goals, this indicates a high service quality. Instructors can help by dividing the main goal (e.g., to lose a certain amount of weight) into subgoals so that customers can track their progress step by step and maintain their motivation.

The outcome embraces the results of the process. The main task is the fulfilment of expected benefits, not the service itself (Ko and Pastore 2004). In particular, instructors should emphasise workout-related outcomes. Customers purchase fitness services and subscribe to memberships because of existing problems: They want to improve their fitness level, lose weight or feel healthier. If they are unable to fulfil these objectives, they are likely to quit (Brehm and Eberhardt 1995; Rampf 1999).

Communicating About the Characteristics of Fitness Services

Because fitness services differ from other service industries in that its process is characterised by collective influences, physical exertion and intimacy, fitness instructors must have excellent communication skills.

Group Dynamics Affecting Service Perception

Whether working out on equipment or participating in group lessons, customers of fitness clubs are constantly surrounded by other clients.

Fitness services have more or less the character of collective services, because the level of interaction among club members is relatively high (Ko and Pastore 2004). The perception of service quality within the workout session of customer A, who is currently using the leg press, can be strongly affected by the behaviour of both customer B, who is sitting at the chest press machine and the outfit of customer C, who is lying on the leg curler nearby. Instructors must use their communication skills to demonstrate that they are completely focused on the needs of each customer. They must listen well, exhibit empathy and adjust nonverbal communication, like positive body language or eye contact. These communication aspects help to reduce the possible negative influences of the group dynamic and strengthen the client's feeling of individuality.

Physical Exertion

When people subscribe to a membership at a fitness centre, they decide to pay money for physical exertion. They do not pay for a comfortable product that allows them to relax and consume something passively. If they want to achieve physical improvements, they must pursue a demanding workout schedule wherein they burn calories, develop muscles and focus their concentration. Losing weight, increasing strength or improving mental well-being are all goals of different exercise customers. Fitness training centres offer the perfect conditions for attaining success, but customers will not achieve their goals if they are not willing to experience physical exertion. For high-quality service, instructors must convince customers that regular workouts in the gym are as necessary as daily dental care.

Without the assistance of an instructor, the likelihood of customers cancelling their membership is high. Instructors must steadfastly convince customers that following a regular workout schedule in a fitness centre is the central premise for receiving physical benefits, and that it offers more benefits than a cheaper or even free activity like jogging can provide. Thus, instructors need exceptional communication skills in order to maintain the customer's motivation. Instructors who exhibit self-confidence and professionalism can successfully motivate their customers. They must also set a positive example with regard to their workout habits.

Intimacy

As compared to other services (figure 1.2), fitness services are very intimate. Instructors deal with the bodies and health of their custom-

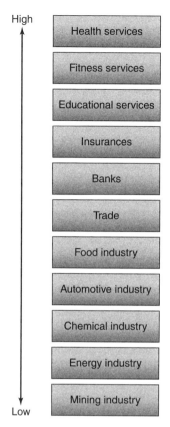

High

Health services

Fitness services

Educational services

Insurances

Banks

Trade

Food industry

Automotive industry

Chemical industry

Energy industry

Mining industry

Low

Figure 1.2 Level of service intimacy.

Adapted from Zollner 1995.

ers. This requires sensitivity in communication. Instructors should pay attention to their personal habits, such as clothing choice, haircut and cleanliness, in order to demonstrate professionalism for services that entail high intimacy (Eckmann 2007).

Successful Customers Are Loyal Customers

The main purpose of exercise for customers is to improve their physical or mental condition. By analysing the reasons that members cancel their memberships in greater detail, it becomes obvious that workouts and customer service have a strong impact: Customers cancel because they do not achieve their workout aims or because they feel poorly supervised or unsatisfied with their general workout assistance (Brehm and Eberhardt 1995; Rampf 1999). A majority of the identified deficits relate to the process or outcome orientation. The consequences are serious: Customers who do not achieve their goals are unsatisfied, and they may quit. These unsatisfied customers may spread negative word-of-mouth propaganda about the fitness centre. In contrast, a successful and satisfied customer is a valuable element for marketing.

No matter how empathetic and pleasant the instructors are, without a professional system for managing customer relationships, which observes the customers' achievement of workout-related goals and subgoals, a fitness centre's service cannot be customer oriented. Additionally, instructors must be aware that other issues like unhealthy lifestyle or nutrition can threaten customers' ability to achieve their goals, and thus threaten the perceived success of the centre's fitness services. The aforementioned system should include the following phases:

1. Assessment (health check, case history)
2. Objectives (primary goal, subgoals)
3. Schedule (measures, planning)
4. Training (implementation, accompaniment, optimisation)
5. Evaluation (achievement of goals, measurement of satisfaction)

Managing Conflicts and Unsatisfied Customers

When customers openly communicate their dissatisfaction, instructors and managers must interpret this as an opportunity to adjust their service behaviour, because dissatisfied customers often quit without supplying any information. Unhappy customers can be converted into happy customers if every complaint is taken seriously. Once again, here, empathy plays an important role. However, empathy can only work if employees are empowered to intervene. Instructors must be allowed by fitness centre management to react quickly to complaints. Often, customers want to be heard and understood (Eckmann 2007). With a professional workout-related management system, the systematic management of complaints can compensate for customer dissatisfaction and reduce the fluctuation rate (see figure 1.3).

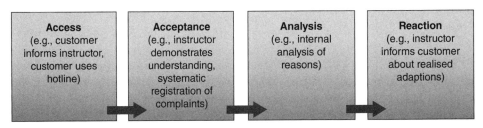

Figure 1.3 Steps of complaint management.
Adapted from Stauss and Seidel 2007.

Conclusion

Regarding the relationship between customer services and customer orientation and bearing in mind the approach of Meffert and Bruhn (2008), customer service has to be implemented in all three phases of the service chain (potential, process and outcome orientation). Although many organisations still emphasise the first phase, considering the essentials of this chapter, the most important elements of customer service are connected with concrete service delivery. Concrete service delivery refers to all the aspects in one-to-one situations and the outcome of this process: customers who achieve their training goals. A service-oriented instructor knows the expectations of the customer, transfers these expectations into necessary characteristics of the service process and always monitors the results of the training process. Further, disruptive factors like group dynamics and physical exertion must be considered during service delivery. Finally, high-quality fitness service can be achieved only by referring to the advice of Scharnbacher and Kiefer: 'Be clean and well organised, react flexibly and show confidence. Appreciate the wishes of the customers and demonstrate that you are reliable. Keep promises you have given' (2003, p. 73).

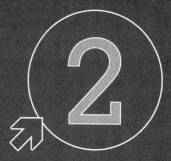

Communication: Giving and Gaining Feedback

Vera Simões

Rita Santos Rocha

The instructor's communication skills highly influence the quality of intervention in fitness context. Very often the instructors focus the emphasis in their intervention on the technical aspects, masking the importance of knowing how to communicate and how to use behaviours that retain the clients and satisfy their needs. This chapter focuses on the importance of communication in teaching and retaining clients, as well as in giving and receiving feedback.

Role of Communication in Teaching

Teaching is a complex activity that requires instructors to make decisions proactively, plan sessions and interact with participants and clients. The primary goal of an instructor or teacher must be for the participants to learn motor skills and improve their performance (Murcia and Oliveira 2002). Regardless of the context in which instructors are acting, they should provide the conditions that increase their participants' motor skill level and help them achieve realistic goals. In order to do so, it is crucial that instructors know how to intervene pedagogically, use appropriate strategies to individualise learning, diagnose problems, guide the class and correct mistakes (Franco 2002). With appropriate communication and strong leadership, fitness instructors can help participants learn new behaviours and modify existing ones (Sarmento 2004). This author states that 'the pedagogical act should not happen randomly, it must be thought, reflected and should be a result of a rational process, supported by principles, purposes and goals' (Sarmento 2004, p. 71).

Communication assumes a prominent role in effective teaching (Castañer et al. 2010) and promotes interpersonal relationships. In the context of sport, Silva and Beresford (2004) write that communication often makes the difference between success and failure.

Appropriate communication and instruction are fundamental skills that instructors must master in order to be effective (Kennedy and Yoke 2005). In order to better understand these processes, we must reflect about instructors' professional activity, particularly about their learning and teaching techniques.

Importance of Communication in Teaching and Retaining Clients

According to Knop (2004) the quality of service is the factor that most contributes to the success of a fitness club. One of the most important sources of competitive advantage for an organisation is its human resources. Attracting new clients and retaining existing ones are fundamental to the success of any fitness club, both of which particularly depend on human resources (Woo and Chelladurai 2012). Fitness instructors have a very important and active role in this process (Papadimitriou and Karteroliotis 2000).

Recently, Fernández, Carrión and Ruiz (2012) performed a study with 7,000 clients of fitness clubs. In their report they conclude from participant feedback that human resources is the variable that best indicates the quality of the clubs, and that human resources are directly related to participant satisfaction levels. These results are far more important, since clients' overall satisfaction with a service is directly related to their loyalty (Pedragosa and Correia 2009). In a study involving 184 fitness participants, Bodet (2006) concludes that the behaviour of instructors is the variable that most contributes to client satisfaction.

Considering this, during sessions, instructors should adapt their behaviour to meet the needs of their participants (Franco and Simões 2006). Instructors should periodically evaluate their level of intervention and adjust their performance as necessary (Rinne and Toropainen 1998).

Giving and Gaining Feedback
During Fitness Sessions

Giving feedback is an essential skill that the fitness instructor (whether a coach, personal trainer, or teacher) should take into consideration, since this process is a key factor in facilitating clients' motor learning (Chin 2005) and correcting or modifying their performance.

The behaviours of coaches, personal trainers, and fitness instructors influence the development of their athletes or participants. Effective professionals use frequent feedback, with the primary objective of teaching, correcting and motivating athletes or participants (Côté and Sedgwick 2003; Franco and Simões 2006). In a study by Franco and Simões (2006) fitness participants preferred that their instructors use encouragement, give feedback while they were performing exercises (not afterwards), use a combination of verbal feedback and gestures (rather than kinaesthetic feedback), inform them how to perform the exercises correctly using spoken affirmations and accompany them throughout the correction processes (observe the participant's performance, give feedback, observe it again and then give more feedback) instead of giving feedback and then leaving to observe another participant. Côté and Sedgwick (2003) cite several studies that indicate that effective coaches often provide high levels of correction and instruction. Alternatively, Molinero, Salguero, Tabernero, Tuero, and Marquez (2005) suggest that fitness instructors follow a certain number of guidelines in order to reduce the dropout rate in physical activity, particularly about giving feedback during physical activity.

Characteristics of Feedback
During Fitness Sessions

Feedback has various functions, including reinforcing behaviours and providing information and motivation (Young and King 2000). Essentially, the instructor's feedback must help participants understand the motor learning process. The feedback that participants give their instructor is also very important for adjusting teaching behaviour. Thus, feedback may also facilitate reinforcement like a sanction or a reward. Feedback is considered a key variable for successful learning (Gusthart et al. 1997).

Feedback is the point of connection between two complementary phenomena: learning and teaching (Piéron 1999). This pedagogical action is assumed as a personal relationship between teacher and student (Piéron 1996) or instructor and client. For this author, feedback results from a set of actions taken by the instructor, including observing and identifying errors, making the decision to react or not, determining the nature and cause of the error and intervening and following up on the reaction, i.e., the results in behaviour after receiving feedback (Piéron 1996).

Some factors related to effective performance of fitness instructors and coaches include the competence to diagnose technical errors and prescribe solutions, as well as the knowledge of how to correct errors (Rosado et al. 2004). This capability is known as *pedagogical feedback*. Another way of understanding feedback is that, during the performance of a cognitive or motor task, participants receive certain types of information, provided largely by the instructor, which they can use to improve or correct their motor tasks and thus improve their performance (Seibert and Francis 2000). Abraham and Collins (2006) interviewed elite sport coaches and found that the coaches identified the power of supplying feedback to the athletes as one of the key elements of sport pedagogy. Rosado et al. (2004) go further and state that the value of feedback from coaches, among the effective solutions they propose, depends on the observations they make about the motor performance, as well as on their competency in detecting errors, determining their causes and then prioritising a process of resolution. These authors reinforce the importance of giving greater attention to the issue of *feedback competency*, where the feedback seems to be essential for learning to occur. Also, it is important to further the study on the role of the feedback (Benda 2006). According to Piéron (1999), studying and analysing what happens in a classroom and observing the behaviours of teachers and their students, as well as the relationships between them, are fundamental to improving the teaching and learning process. The same should happen during a fitness workout. The systematic observation becomes an essential tool for this purpose, constituting itself as a method of data collection aimed towards accurately representing reality. The need to supervise the fitness professionals as well as gather information about their behaviour through direct and systematic observation in real situations and contexts are determining factors for the success of the educational process (Sarmento 2004; Simões and Santos-Rocha 2013). More information for practical intervention is provided in *EuropeActive's Foundations for Exercise Professionals* (Simões and Santos-Rocha 2015/in press).

Conclusion

Effective communication, including appropriate feedback, is essential for fitness instructors. It's important that instructors are aware of the importance of having effective communication and appropriate feedback as tools for teaching and retaining clients. It's also important that the technical directors of fitness clubs look into the issue of communication and feedback and in their plans of action implement strategies, preparation and reflection sessions, which allow its instructors to improve and optimize their behaviors during the sessions. Training providers in fitness areas, in their study plans, should contemplate these issues in order to teach and help instructors act in accordance with the client's needs.

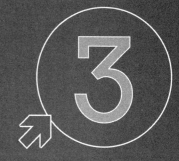

Cardiorespiratory Exercise

Paolo Benvenuti

Silvano Zanuso

For participants in fitness programmes, the ability of the lungs to provide oxygen to the blood and of the heart and circulatory system to transport blood and its nutrients to the body's tissue are crucial. Fitness instructors must understand these basic physiological concepts, and they should be able to apply each component of a cardiorespiratory exercise programme: leading the warm-up and cool-down; monitoring the mode, frequency and duration of exercise; and providing the information and guidance necessary to ensure client's safety. Moreover fitness instructors can choose from a number of training methods and cardiorespiratory activities when offering suggestions to clients in order to meet their different needs. This chapter provides basic information on the mechanism of cardiorespiratory exercises, as well as on the benefits of participation and different teaching methodologies.

Cardiovascular Response to Exercise

The human body requires a constant supply of energy in order to carry out its many functions. This energy comes from two main metabolic processes: anaerobic and aerobic metabolism. Anaerobic metabolism is used for short, high-intensity exercises because the accumulated lactic acid quickly tires the muscles. Aerobic metabolism meets the demand for energy in most low- or medium-intensity cardiorespiratory exercises. Here, exercisers can work longer because lactic acid is produced at a lower rate, which means it can be more easily metabolised by the body. A well-designed exercise programme enhances the capabilities of those metabolic processes and improves the body's overall functionality.

To understand cardiorespiratory exercises (which involve the cardiovascular and respiratory systems), we need to clarify some terms. In *cardiovascular, cardio* stands for heart and *vascular* stands for the circulatory system. The cardiovascular system includes the heart, with its four chambers; arteries, in which blood moves away from the heart; veins, in which blood returns to the heart; and a system of capillaries, which transport blood between small arteries and small veins. In exercise physiology, fitness work that involves the heart and lungs is termed *cardiorespiratory exercise*. In this case the word *respiratory* stands for the respiratory system. Cardiorespiratory exercises also improve the body's ability to transport oxygen to the working muscles. Figure 3.1 separates the two halves of the heart to better illustrate the functions of the heart's right and left sides.

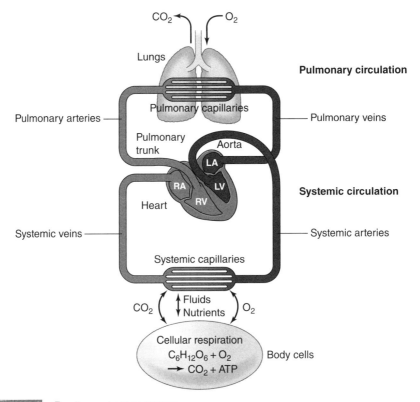

Figure 3.1 Cardiorespiratory system.

Reprinted, by permission, from D. Smith, 2011, *Advanced cardiovascular exercise physiology* (Champaign, IL: Human Kinetics), 4.

Before examining in detail what happens at the cardiovascular level as a result of training, it is useful to point out the meaning of the following two terms, which indicate more or less persistent changes of a body function:

- Acute responses or *adjustments*: rapid but temporary modifications that result from a single exercise.
- Chronic responses or *adaptations*: changes in a function or a structure of the body as a result of repeated or chronic exercise.

Effective training often consists simply of a number of adaptations involving both physical and psychological dimensions that are advantageous for global wellness.

The benefits of cardiorespiratory activity are tied to adaptations involving the entire oxygen transport system.

Acute Responses or Adjustments

Moving from rest to maximal physical exertion substantially increases energy requirements. For that reason adenosine triphosphate (ATP), which provides energy only for several seconds, needs to be constantly resynthesised. To constantly deliver energy to the working muscles the body relies on the respiratory and cardiovascular systems to provide oxygen and nutrients and remove waste products.

To produce ATP the aerobic system requires sufficient oxygen and uses glycogen, fat and protein as energy substrates. The relative contributions of aerobic and anaerobic (which rapidly provides ATP for a limited time) metabolism depend on oxygen consumption (related to respiration), delivery (related to cardiovascular activity) and use (related to the capacity of muscles to extract oxygen). These activities are commensurate with the energy demand of a given exercise.

The acute responses of exercise encompass both cardiorespiratory and circulatory functions to support the increased oxygen demands of the working muscles. Delivering oxygenated blood to muscles during exercise requires acute modifications in heart rate, stroke volume, cardiac output, blood flow, arteriovenous oxygen difference, blood pressure and pulmonary ventilation.

Heart Rate (HR)

As exercise intensity increases, heart rate (HR) also goes up, correlating with both the workload (e.g., the running speed or the resistance on a stationary bike) and the oxygen uptake. The increase in HR response depends on various factors: age, training level, type of activity, body position, medications, total blood volume and environmental factors such as temperature and humidity. The maximal attainable HR decreases with age. Various equations (table 3.1) may

Table 3.1   Equations to Predict Maximal Heart Rate

Name	Equations	Source
Fox	HRmax = 220 − age	Fox S.M., Naughton J.P., Haskell W.L. Physical activity and the prevention of coronary heart disease. *Ann. Clin. Res.* 3: 404–432, 1971.
Tanaka	HRmax = 208 − (0.7 × age)	Tanaka H., Monahan K.D., Seals D.R. Age-predicted maximal heart rate revisited. *J. Am. Coll. Cardiol.* 37: 153–156, 2001.
Gellish	HRmax = 207 − (0.7 × age)	Gellish R.L., Goslin B.R., Olson R.E., McDonald A., Russi G.D., Moudgil V.K. Longitudinal modeling of the relationship between age and maximal heart rate. *Med. Sci. Sports Exerc.* 39: 822–829, 2007.

help instructors estimate this value without administering maximal exercise tests.

Stroke Volume

Stroke volume (SV) is the volume of blood pumped from one ventricle of the heart with each beat. It depends on the capacity of the ventricle to fill with blood during the diastolic phase and to contract during the systolic phase. During exercise, SV increases with exercise intensity (expressed as workload) until 50 percent of aerobic capacity, where it nearly reaches its maximum. After that point, it increases only slightly.

Cardiac Output

Cardiac output (CO) is the volume of blood pumped by the heart within one minute; thus it is the product of SV and HR. In healthy individuals CO increases linearly with exercise intensity (expressed as workload) from a value at rest of approximately 5 litres per minute to a maximum of about 20 litres per minute. Maximum values of CO response depend on various factors, including age, training level, type of activity (body posture) and medications. At exercise intensities higher than 50 percent of $\dot{V}O_2$max, the increase in CO results solely from the continued rise in HR.

Blood Flow

Exercise changes the distribution of blood flow. At rest, only 15 to 20 percent of the cardiac output goes to the muscles; the remainder goes to visceral organs, the heart and the brain. During exercise there is an enormous increase in blood flow to the working muscles (up to 90 percent) and the heart (myocardial blood flow increases up to five times); blood supply to the brain is maintained at resting levels, whilst there is a significant decrease in blood flow to internal organs (e.g., the liver and kidneys).

Arteriovenous Oxygen Difference

The difference between the oxygen contained in blood located in the arteries (arterial blood) and that contained in the veins (venous blood) is called the *arteriovenous oxygen difference*. At rest this difference is about 5 millilitres of oxygen per decilitre of blood, yielding a coefficient of oxygen utilisation of 25 percent. During maximal exercise the oxygen content of venous blood decreases significantly, increasing the arteriovenous difference from 5 to 15 millilitres of oxygen per decilitre of blood, yielding a coefficient of oxygen utilisation that reaches 75 percent.

Blood Pressure

Blood pressure (BP) is the parameter that shows a linear increase with exercise intensity (expressed as workload). Maximal values can reach up to 220 torrs (mmHg). Diastolic BP typically remains unchanged (or decreases only slightly); thus the difference between systolic and diastolic blood pressure (pulse pressure) increases linearly with exercise intensity.

Pulmonary Ventilation

Pulmonary ventilation ($\dot{V}_E$) is the parameter that expresses the volume of air exchanged per minute. $\dot{V}_E$ for a sedentary man at rest is about 6 litres per minute. At maximal exertion this value can reach up to 150 litres per minute. During moderate exercise $\dot{V}_E$ increases thanks to an increase of the tidal volume (normal volume of air displaced between normal inspiration and expiration when extra effort is not applied), whilst during vigorous exercise $\dot{V}_E$ increases mainly because of respiratory rate. A linear relation exists between $\dot{V}_E$ and oxygen consumption and carbon dioxide production. However, at critical exercise intensity, $\dot{V}_E$ increases disproportionally in relation to $\dot{V}O_2$, leading to an increase of serum lactate production and $\dot{V}CO_2$. Ventilation does not normally limit aerobic capacity.

Chronic Responses or Adaptations

When an exercise stimulus is constantly repeated over time, it becomes a chronic stimulus that provides beneficial permanent adaptations. A large body of literature now demonstrates that well-designed aerobic programmes can lead to significant improvements in aerobic capacity (expressed as increases in $\dot{V}O_2$max), with the greatest benefits achieved by people with the lowest fitness levels. Since at any given workload the metabolic requirement (oxygen consumption) is similar across different fitness levels, less-fit subjects have improved their aerobic capacity by working at a lower percentage of their $\dot{V}O_2$max; for that reason, all people can improve their aerobic capacity, regardless of age and health status. Improving aerobic capacity offers some protection against cardiovascular mortality and enhances the ability to perform activities of daily living. Increases in aerobic capacity can also be attributed to cardiovascular and cardiorespiratory changes.

Heart Rate

Heart rate plays a fundamental role in delivering oxygen to the working muscles. After repeated exposure to aerobic training stimuli, resting HR generally decreases. This reduction seems to be more evident in subjects who were previously unconditioned. Resting HR is restrained by the vagus nerve, and vagal tone appears to increase during rest, leading to a decreased resting heart rate of approximately 10 to 15 beats per minute. After aerobic conditioning, maximal heart rate is unchanged or slightly decreased (3 to 10 beats per minute).

Stroke Volume

As a result of chronic aerobic training, SV increases secondary to an improved contractile capacity thanks to an enhanced mechanical ability of myocardial fibres to produce force and to an increase in venous return (Frank-Starling mechanism). The increased SV obtained through chronic aerobic training allows individuals to exercise at similar workloads but at a lower heart rate, thus decreasing the oxygen demand at the myocardial level.

Cardiac Output

This parameter, which is strictly correlated to stroke volume, is significantly higher in subjects exposed to chronic aerobic exercise when compared with sedentary individuals. At any given workload CO is similar across different fitness levels and before and after training.

Arteriovenous Oxygen Difference

Individuals who are exposed to chronic aerobic training enhance their ability to extract the oxygen that is transported in circulating blood. As a result, an increase in oxygen consumption can be obtained, determined by a higher arteriovenous oxygen difference. However, since conditioned individuals have a greater ability to use oxygen at the cellular level, at the submaximal level, the arteriovenous oxygen difference is similar between trained and untrained subjects. This parameter is significantly greater in trained subjects only when its value is close to that of VO_2max.

Blood Pressure

Recent evidence shows that in hypertensive, prehypertensive and normotensive adults, aerobic exercise yields important reductions in systolic and diastolic BP. In regard to systolic BP, the result of aerobic training is that at any fixed submaximal workload, trained subjects show generally lower systolic BP than untrained subjects do. In terms of training level, systolic BP is lower in trained subjects than in untrained subjects.

Blood Lactate

Lactic acid, or lactate, is a by-product of anaerobic glycolysis. During aerobic exercise it is associated with the onset of significant anaerobic contribution to exercise metabolism. During aerobic exercise executed at submaximal intensities, blood lactate is buffered to maintain a tolerable acid–base balance. When its production exceeds the buffering capacity of the metabolic system, fatigue rapidly increases, leading to exercise termination. Endurance exercises, which improve the oxidative capacity of skeletal muscle, lead trained individuals to have lower lactate levels at any fixed submaximal work rate since they produce less and buffer more of the lactic acid produced.

Pulmonary Ventilation

As stated before, ventilation generally does not limit exercise in healthy individuals, and it is either unaffected or only modestly affected by aerobic training. Although exercise training may increase maximal ventilatory capacity, it is unclear whether it provides any advantage other than increasing the buffering capacity for lactate.

Warm-Up and Cool-Down

To ensure safety and a positive training experience, before participants start any cardiorespiratory activity, instructors should help them gradually prepare their bodies for the increased physiological demands involved in the training routine. The following section lists the physiological reasons to warm up and cool down before and after exercise. Table 3.2 provides examples of warm-up and cool-down activities for different types of exercise.

Table 3.2   Activity-Specific Warm-Up and Cool-Down Activities

Primary conditioning exercise	Warm-up and cool-down activities
Dance aerobics and step	Graduated low-level aerobic activity utilising the same muscle groups
Jogging and running	Walking, light jogging
Sprinting	Jogging and running at a graduated pace in intervals
Outdoor cycling	Begin with relatively flat terrain in lower gears; gradually shift to higher gears and steeper terrain
Stationary cycling	Start cycling against little or no resistance at 2/3 of the pedal crank rpm used in the conditioning phase
Stationary exercise device	Begin with 50–60% of intended conditioning workload or speed; the duration of the submaximal graduated warm-up should be proportional to the peak intensity of the conditioning workload
Rope skipping	Power-walking or rope skipping at slow pace
Competitive tennis	Light jogging or volleying at a graduated tempo that is proportional to the level of the game
Lap swimming	Begin with a slow crawl and gradually increase arm stroke and pace, or begin with 1 or 2 slow laps

Adapted from *ACE personal trainer manual* 1997.

Benefits of a Proper Warm-Up

A proper warm-up increases the blood flow to the working muscles and confers many other benefits:

- **Increases muscle temperature.** The temperature increases within muscles that are used during a warm-up routine. A warmed muscle both contracts more forcefully and relaxes more quickly. Also, it reduces the probability of overstretching a muscle and causing injury.

- **Increases body temperature.** This improves muscle elasticity, also reducing the risk of strains and pulls.

- **Dilates blood vessels.** This reduces the resistance to blood flow and lowers stress on the heart.

- **Improves cooling mechanisms.** By activating the heat-dissipation mechanisms in the body (efficient sweating) a person can cool efficiently and help prevent overheating early in the event or race.

- **Increases blood temperature.** The temperature of blood increases as it travels through the muscles. As blood tempera-

Physiological and Psychological Reasons to Warm Up and Cool Down

Warming up does the following:

- Permits a gradual increase in metabolic requirement (e.g., oxygen consumption), which enhances cardiorespiratory performance (e.g., a higher maximum cardiac output and oxygen consumption)
- Prevents the premature onset of blood lactic acid accumulation and fatigue in higher-level aerobic exercise
- Causes a maximal increase in muscle temperature, which reduces the likelihood of muscle injury
- Facilitates neural transmission
- Increases coronary blood flow in early stages of the conditioning exercise, lessening the potential for myocardial ischemia
- Provides a screening mechanism for the potential musculoskeletal or metabolic problems that may increase at higher intensities
- Provides psychological preparation for higher levels of work (i.e., increases arousal and focus on exercise)

Cooling down does the following:

- Prevents postexercise venous blood pooling and extreme drops in blood pressure, thereby reducing the likelihood of postexercise light-headedness or fainting
- Reduces the immediate postexercise tendency for muscles to spasm or cramp
- Reduces the concentration of exercise hormones (e.g., norepinephrine) that are at relatively high levels immediately after vigorous aerobic exercise. This reduction will lower the probability of postexercise disturbance in cardiac rhythm. (Giese 1988; McArdle and Katch 1996).

ture rises, the binding of oxygen to haemoglobin weakens so oxygen is more readily available to working muscles, which may improve endurance.

- **Improves range of motion.** This reduces muscular-articular injuries.
- **Facilitates hormonal changes.** The body increases its production of the hormones responsible for regulating energy production. During the warm-up this balance of hormones makes more carbohydrates and fatty acids available for energy production.
- **Aids mental preparation.** The warm-up is a good time to mentally prepare for the training by clearing the mind of distractions and increasing focus. Positive imagery can also help participants relax and build concentration.

Typical Warm-Up Exercises

Low-level aerobic exercise is essential for maximising safety and economy of movement during the subsequent aerobic training. The warm-up should increase heart rate, blood pressure, oxygen consumption and flexibility of the target muscles in a progressive way. The ideal warm-up should consist of two components—graduated aerobic movements and flexibility exercises.

Graduated Aerobic Movements

These movements are executed either on machines (e.g., treadmills or stationary bikes) or without machines (e.g., jogging, slow-tempo aerobic movements). The warm-up procedure should provide a graduated level of activity similar to the primary conditioning activity, but movements should be executed at an intensity well below that of the primary conditioning activity. The length of the warm-up depends on the duration of the main activity and the participant's conditioning level.

Flexibility Exercises

Flexibility exercises should be related to the main activity participants will perform during the session (e.g., stretching of the rotator cuff before a session on a rowing machine or stretching of calf and hamstrings prior to running). To avoid injury the best time to stretch a muscle is after blood flow and temperature have increased. Stretching a cold muscle can increase the risk of injury from pulls and tears. So it is better to perform gradual aerobic exercise before stretching. Instructors should make sure the warm-up begins gradually and uses the muscles that will be stressed during exercise. They should keep in mind that participants should also stretch after exercise when their muscles are warm and pliable from increased blood flow.

Cool-Down

Each exercise session should terminate with a cool-down with the purpose of slowly decreasing the load of the cardiorespiratory apparatuses that have been elevated during training. Low-level aerobic exercises such as walking, jogging or cycling with low resistance are recommended. Cooling down helps restore normal circulation and prevent post-exercise fainting and dizziness and the sudden pooling of blood in the veins. For subjects at high cardiovascular risk, a gradual decrease in the intensity of exercise is crucial; in fact because stress hormones are released during exercise (e.g., adrenalin), sudden cessation of the workout without a proper cool-down may adversely affect cardiac function. Normally, 5 to 10 minutes of cool-down are sufficient. The aerobic component of the cool-down should be followed by some stretching of the muscle groups that were active during training.

Modifications to Allow for Individual Differences

To be safe, effective and individualised, a cardiorespiratory exercise programme must consider the major factors that relate to exercise response and must have specific instructions. The most updated guidelines on effectiveness and safety can be found in the American College of Sports Medicine's position stands (Garber et al. 2011). The factors related to exercise improvements include initial fitness level and exercise intensity, duration, frequency and mode.

Exercise Intensity

Intensity refers both to the external workload (e.g., speed on a treadmill or resistance on a stationary bike) and the internal load (e.g., heart rate or $\dot{V}O_2$). Thus, intensity can be considered either in absolute or relative terms. If two different participants are doing the same workload at the same rate (e.g., 5 kilometres per hour on a treadmill), they are exercising at the same *absolute intensity*. However, even though they are exercising with the same absolute intensity, a considerable effort for one subject could be very light for a well-conditioned person. For this reason, exercises are also classified and prescribed in terms of *relative intensity*. The basic measures of relative intensity for instructors to use include HR, heart rate reserve (HRR), and oxygen consumption ($\dot{V}O_2$) (table 3.3). Generally, to establish training intensity, either maximum HR or $\dot{V}O_2$ are measured or estimated, and then a training load is assigned based on percentages of those maximums.

Table 3.3   Relationship Between Heart Rate Reserve (HRR), Oxygen Consumption ($\dot{V}O_2$), and Maximal Heart Rate (HRmax)

Percent HRR/$\dot{V}O_2$	Percent HRmax
28	50
42	60
56	70
70	80
83	90
100	100

McArdle and Katch 1996.

Exercise Duration

Even though the ideal duration for optimal cardiorespiratory improvement has not been identified, to gain significant benefits, the conditioning period of aerobic training should vary from approximately 15 to 60 minutes. The duration depends on exercise intensity: With high-intensity training, improvements can be obtained even with 10 minutes of work, whilst more than 30 minutes of continuous exercise may be required to produce training effects at low intensities. The overall conditioning response to an aerobic exercise programme is the result of the intensity and the duration of exercise; instructors must carefully manage those variables according to the subjective characteristics of each client.

Exercise Frequency

There is not a clear answer on how many days of training per week are best for obtaining significant benefits. The ideal frequency of exercise probably depends on the duration, the intensity and, more importantly, on the final goal (especially for athletes). However, for the general population, the ACSM recommends three to five days of training per week, with no more than two days off between sessions, to both improve cardiorespiratory fitness and maintain body fat at a near optimum level.

Initial Fitness Level

The amount of improvement experienced from training is related to the initial fitness level of the participant: The lower the starting level, the greater the possible improvements. If participants' initial capacity is already high, they will experience relatively little improvement. Obviously an improvement of 5 percent in physiological function and performance of an elite athlete is just as important as a 30 percent increase for a sedentary person. Also, the lower the initial fitness level, the more rapid the improvement. For participants with poor fitness levels, just three weeks of training can lead to significant benefits. On the other hand they can quickly lose those benefits if they suddenly stop training.

Exercise Mode

As long as training involves large muscle groups in an aerobic rhythmic fashion, and intensity, duration and frequency are held constant, participants experience similar training improvements regardless of training mode. The ideal exercise programme for healthy subjects should encompass different exercise modes: walking, running, bicycling and swimming. Obviously individuals trained on a cycle ergometer will show greater improvements when tested on this ergometer than on a treadmill. Likewise those training by running will show the highest improvements when tested on a treadmill.

Cardiorespiratory Training Methods

With aerobic endurance training, the body becomes better able to produce ATP through aerobic metabolism. The cardiorespiratory and aerobic energy systems become more efficient at delivering oxygen to the working muscles and converting carbohydrate and fat to energy. Many different ways of training improve aerobic endurance. The duration, frequency and intensity of each type of training vary, and focusing on slightly different energy systems and skills will result in different physical adaptations. The training must be designed to provide sufficient cardiovascular overload for stimulating increases in stroke volume and cardiac output. Both brief bouts of repeated exercise (interval training) as well as continuous, long-duration exercise (continuous training) and Fartlek training through a systematic overload of the aerobic system can improve aerobic capacity. Some of the most well-known cardiorespiratory training programmes include continuous training, interval training and Fartlek training.

Continuous Training

This type of training is the most common type of endurance training. It serves as the foundation for marathon runners, long-distance cyclists and participants in other sports that demand long and sustained energy outputs. It is also the easiest form of endurance training for new or novice exercisers. It involves steady-state exercises performed at either moderate or high aerobic exercise intensity, (e.g., 56 percent HRR/$\dot{V}O_2$ or 70 percent HRmax) for a duration typically exceeding 20 minutes. Instructors use different methods to establish whether participants have entered the training zone such as a specific test (either maximal or submaximal), a given percentage of predicted maximal heart rate or rate of subjective perceived exertion. Continuous training is submaximal in nature; therefore it can be sustained for a considerable length of time. Typically the overload is obtained by increasing the duration of the exercise, even though the intensity can also be manipulated. Considering that high-intensity training could be potentially hazardous for subjects with some chronic conditions (especially for those with cardiovascular diseases), continuous training is particularly suitable for those approaching a training programme. When applied to sport, continuous training executed for very long durations allows the largest aerobic adaptations in both central circulation and peripheral tissue.

Interval Training

This type of training consists of short, repeated, but intense physical efforts (3 to 5 minutes of exercise followed by short rest periods). The repeated exercise bouts (with resting intervals) can vary from a few seconds to several minutes, depending on the training goal. The variables that contribute to determining the different effects of this type of training are basically the intensity and duration of the exercise bouts and the number and duration of the intervals. Modifications of any of these variables can be made to meet different training purposes: Longer exercise bouts improve the aerobic system whilst shorter bouts place emphasis on the anaerobic energy system. The basic advantage of interval training is that it permits participants to perform high-intensity exercise for a relatively long period of time. Thus, a normally exhausting high-intensity training volume can be achieved by balancing exercise bouts and resting periods.

Fartlek Training

Fartlek training combines some or all of the other training methods during a long, moderate-intensity training session. With Fartlek, participants run at alternating fast and slow speeds on a course with both flat and hilly terrain. This training does not include precise manipulation of the intensity and the duration of exercise bouts and rests; the overall training intensity is determined by both the physical characteristics of the course and the subjective sensations of the performer. Fartlek training is considered ideal for general conditioning and for off-season training, and it provides a certain freedom and variety in the workouts.

Dose–Response Relationship Based on Evidence

For instructors who design exercise programmes, fitting exercise into a busy daily schedule of a client is often a challenge. Making time to move each day is important, but how much is enough? Thirty minutes a day? An hour a day? Three sessions of 45 minutes a week? There is no single answer to this question; it depends essentially on the objective of the physical activity or exercise programme (e.g., general health benefits, physical fitness or specific performance goals) and on some specific questions such as minimum duration and type of activities. However, instructors should know these generic but evidence-based guidelines.

General Health Benefits

The American College of Sports Medicine (ACSM) and U.S. Centers for Disease Control and Prevention (CDC) have made the valid and long-standing recommendations that health gains can come from as little as 30 minutes of moderate-intensity physical activity most days of the week, with workouts of greater duration and intensity providing greater health benefits. Additional recent scientific and clinical evidence, summarised in the Physical Activity Advisory Committee Report, has supported the 30-minute recommendation. A prestigious scientific panel of the Institute of Medicine (IOM) also released a report on dietary guidelines that calls for 60 minutes of moderately intense physical activity each day in order to maintain weight.

In the past some media coverage implied that the 30-minute recommendation was incorrect, and should be replaced by the IOM's 60-minute recommendation. This misinterpretation caused many to express concern over the confusion caused by two different exercise recommendations. To eliminate the confusion, the ACSM and other organisations emphasised that the recommendations serve different purposes (30 minutes of physical activity per day are sufficient for gaining some health benefits, and 60 minutes of activity per day may be required for avoiding weight gain).

The report has opened the door for the scientific and clinical communities to further examine the research and evidence of linkages among physical activity, diet and health. But in the interim, with the prevalence of people who get no daily exercise at all, it is important to clarify and reinforce that even small increases in physical activity, as little as 30 minutes per day, can improve health.

However, experts point out that the amount of physical activity required for maximal or optimal health benefits is unknown, and more research is needed to advance our understanding. 'We also are uncertain about the amount of activity necessary to prevent weight gain, and there is extensive individual variation. For example, some individuals never exercise, yet also do not gain any weight over their adult years, while others gain a substantial amount of weight despite daily jogging' (2011 letter from Professor S. Blair to the authors; unreferenced).

Quantity and Quality

The latest ACSM recommendation (Nieman and Swain 2011) represents the most updated and authoritative document answer to this question. The publication clearly states that most adults should engage in moderate-intensity cardiorespiratory exercise training for ≥30 minutes per day on at least five days per week, for a total of at least 150 minutes per week, vigorous-intensity cardiorespiratory exercise training for 20 minutes per day on at least three days per week (≥60 minutes per week), or a combination of moderate- and vigorous-intensity exercise to achieve a total energy expenditure of 500 to 1,000 METs per minutes per week or more. (MET refers to *metabolic equivalent*, and 1 MET is the rate of energy expenditure while sitting at rest. It is taken by convention to be an oxygen uptake of 3.5 millilitres per kilogram of body weight per minute. Physical activities frequently are classified by their intensity, using the MET as a reference.) On two or three days per week, adults should also perform resistance exercises for each of the major muscle groups, as well as neuromotor exercises involving balance, agility and coordination. Crucial to maintaining joint range of movement, completing a series of flexibility exercises for each the major muscle–tendon groups (a total of 60 seconds per exercise) at least two days per week is recommended. The exercise programme should be modified according to an individual's habitual physical activity, physical function, health status, exercise responses and stated goals. Adults who are unable or unwilling to meet the exercise targets outlined here still can benefit from engaging in less exercise than is recommended. In addition to exercising regularly, health benefits can be gained from concurrently reducing total time engaged in sedentary pursuits and interspersing frequent, short bouts of standing and physical activity between periods of sedentary activity, even in physically active adults.

Conclusion

Cardiorespiratory exercise is any type of exercise that increases the work of the heart and lungs over a prolonged period of time. Walking, jogging and running are common forms of cardiorespiratory, or aerobic, exercise.

From running and cycling, to swimming, elliptical cross-training and stepping, the benefits of doing aerobic exercises are numerous and encompass the physiological and psychological domain. The American College of Sports Medicine and the CDC recommend, for health, that adults should accumulate 30 minutes of moderate-intensity physical activity on most days of the week. They recommend 20 to 60 minutes of moderate-intensity physical activity on three to five days per week to improve cardiovascular endurance.

When cardiorespiratory exercises are executed within a fitness and wellness facility, they can be executed for purposes that go beyond health benefits: training for a specific sport, body appearance, weight loss and socialization. No matter the goal of the cardiorespiratory exercise, fitness instructors need to properly understand the basic physiological concepts of aerobic training as well as the different modalities to perform this type of exercise in a safe and effective mode. In this chapter, we have provided the basic information on the mechanism of cardiorespiratory exercises and the benefits of participation and different teaching methodologies.

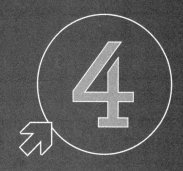

Resistance Exercise

Fernando Naclerio

Jeremy Moody

The potential outcomes achieved by resistance training programme design depend on the relationship between training variables, such as volume, intensity, rest periods, duration and frequency of training, and the mechanical variables, namely selection and type of exercise, in addition to the devices used to provide resistance (Naclerio et al. 2011). Correct exercise technique is a basic but prerequisite requirement of all resistance training programmes, and it is not limited to the level of performance, the programme goal or expected outcomes (Colado and Garcia-Masso 2009). To guide participants through correct exercise technique, instructors must fully understand the limits of the secure range of motion, joint positions that increase the risk of injury (and how to avoid those positions), the training status and history of participants and the technical model of the desired movement.

Evidence accumulated over the last decade has demonstrated that injury risk in resistance training is significantly low compared to other activities such as team sports and gymnastics or fighting sports (Myer et al. 2009). When practiced regularly, following a well-designed programme, resistance training has been shown to be safe and effective (Jones et al. 2000; Myer et al. 2009). The level of safety is maximised when resistance exercises are performed under the supervision of qualified instructors who know how to effectively teach this type of training. Such professionals may provide the most effective interventional approach for reducing the probability of strength training–related injuries, regardless of the age of participants (adults, teenagers or children) (Faigenbaum et al. 2011; Colado and Garcia-Masso 2009). Some authors have made reference to contra-indicated exercises, such as the dead lift or deep squat, that can be performed safely following a sound training process and within the optimal range of motion, volume and intensity and technical ability of the participant (Naclerio and Forte 2011). This chapter focuses on the importance of controlling exercise technique and maintaining correct posture during resistance exercises. It also analyses the mechanisms available for warm-ups and safety recommendations for controlling resistance training exercise. Finally it reviews the dose–response resistance training outcomes for athletes and recreational novice, intermediate and advanced practitioners.

Basic Movement Analysis for Exercise Performance and Technique

Human motion is described in terms of relative anatomical position, as shown in figure 4.1. The sagittal plane divides the body into right and left segments. Movement occurs in a sagittal plane around the transverse or mediolateral axis of rotation and in a front-to-back manner (flexion and extension) and vice versa. The frontal plane divides the body into anterior and posterior regions; thus movement occurs around the anteroposterior axis and in a side-to-side manner (adduction and abduction). The plane occurring around the longitudinal axis is the transverse plane; here the body is split into upper and lower regions, and movement takes place in a horizontal manner (rotation, supination or pronation). Figure 4.2 provides some examples of movements and their respective planes and axes of rotation.

Many human movements and resistance training exercises occur in two or three planes; these may be referred to as multiplanar. The description of movements can be made somewhat more challenging when planes of motion can change depending on the starting position of the exercise or movement. In its simplest form, this basic kinesiological criterion defines a given muscle, for instance, as flexor or extensor on the basis of the torque produced around a single joint; however, the particular nature of body movements creates a complex linked system that uses many joints and segments at any time. This means that muscles that do not cross another joint can still have an effect on movement patterns by the transfer of forces at the active joint (Siff 2004). In the case of isolated exercise, such as the biceps curl, where only one joint is predominantly involved in the action, the traditional approach of movement description could be acceptable,

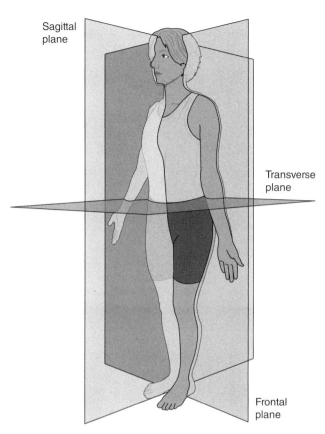

Figure 4.1 Sagittal, frontal and transverse planes and their corresponding axes of rotation in the human body.

Reprinted, by permission, E. Harman, 2008, Biomechanics of resistance exercise. In *Essentials of strength training and conditioning,* 3rd ed., by National Strength and Conditioning Association, edited by T.R. Baechle and R.W. Earle (Champaign, IL: Human Kinetics), 73.

but not if several joints are free to move concurrently in all three planes at the same time. This is the case in the majority of sports movements and resistance training exercises, such as squat or clean, which require the co-ordination and combined force application of a multimuscle and multijoint system. In addition, such a system can act with different or opposite functions throughout the different phases of movement. For instance, during the ascending phase of the squat, extension of the knee and hip occurs simultaneously, so that the quadriceps and hamstring groups are both acting concentrically at the same time. This is because the hamstrings (biceps femoris, semitendinosus and semimembranosus) are technically antagonists of the quadriceps; hence, opposing knee extensor movements occur in this exercise. In the squatting movement however, they behave paradoxically and co-contract with the quadriceps. This synergistic

Wrist—sagittal
Flexion
Exercise: Wrist curl
Sport: Basketball free throw

Extension
Exercise: Wrist extension
Sport: Racquetball backhand

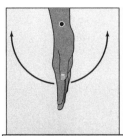

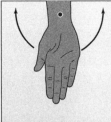

Wrist—frontal
Ulnar deviation
Exercise: Specific wrist curl
Sport: Baseball bat swing

Radial deviation
Exercise: Specific wrist curl
Sport: Golf backswing

Elbow—sagittal
Flexion
Exercise: Biceps curl
Sport: Bowling

Extension
Exercise: Triceps pushdown
Sport: Shot put

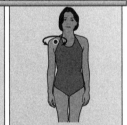

Shoulder—sagittal
Flexion
Exercise: Front shoulder raise
Sport: Boxing uppercut punch

Extension
Exercise: Neutral-grip seated row
Sport: Freestyle swimming stroke

Shoulder—frontal
Adduction
Exercise: Wide-grip lat pulldown
Sport: Swimming breast stroke

Abduction
Exercise: Wide-grip shoulder press
Sport: Springboard diving

Shoulder—transverse
Internal rotation
Exercise: Arm wrestle movement (with dumbbell or cable)
Sport: Baseball pitch

External rotation
Exercise: Reverse arm wrestle movement
Sport: Karate block

Shoulder—transverse
(upper arm to 90° to trunk)
Adduction
Exercise: Dumbbell chest fly
Sport: Tennis forehand

Abduction
Exercise: Bent-over lateral raise
Sport: Tennis backhand

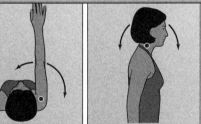

Neck—sagittal
Flexion
Exercise: Neck machine
Sport: Somersault

Extension
Exercise: Dynamic back bridge
Sport: Back flip

Neck—transverse
Left rotation
Exercise: Manual resistance
Sport: Wrestling movement

Right rotation
Exercise: Manual resistance
Sport: Wrestling movement

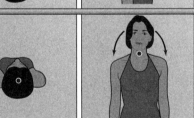

Neck—frontal
Left tilt
Exercise: Neck machine
Sport: Slalom skiing

Right tilt
Exercise: Neck machine
Sport: Slalom skiing

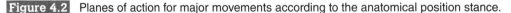

Figure 4.2 Planes of action for major movements according to the anatomical position stance.

Reprinted, by permission, E. Harman, 2008, Biomechanics of resistance exercise. In *Essentials of strength training and conditioning*, 3rd ed., by National Strength and Conditioning Association, edited by T.R. Baechle and R.W. Earle (Champaign, IL: Human Kinetics), 88-89. Adapted from E.A. Harman, M. Johnson, and P.N. Frykman 1992, "A movement-oriented approach to exercise prescription," *NSCA Journal* 14(1): 47-54.

Lower back—sagittal
Flexion
Exercise: Sit-up
Sport: Javelin throw
follow-through

Extension
Exercise: Stiff-leg deadlift
Sport: Back flip

Lower back—transverse
Left rotation
Exercise: Medicine ball side
toss
Sport: Baseball batting

Right rotation
Exercise: Torso machine
Sport: Golf swing

Hip—frontal
Adduction
Exercise: Standing
adduction machine
Sport: Football side step

Abduction
Exercise: Standing
abduction machine
Sport: Rollerblading

Hip—transverse
(upper leg to 90° to trunk)
Adduction
Exercise: Adduction machine
Sport: Karate in-sweep

Abduction
Exercise: Seated abduction
machine
Sport: Wrestling escape

Ankle—sagittal
Dorsiflexion
Exercise: Toe raise
Sport: Running

Plantar flexion
Exercise: Calf (heel) raise
Sport: high jump

Lower back—frontal
Left tilt
Exercise: Medicine ball
overhead hook throw
Sport: Gymnastics side aerial

Right tilt
Exercise: Side bend
Sport: Basketball hook shot

Hip—sagittal
Flexion
Exercise: Leg raise
Sport: American football punt

Extension
Exercise: Back squat
Sport: Long jump take-off

Hip—transverse
Internal rotation
Exercise: Resisted internal rotation
Sport: Basketball pivot movement

External rotation
Exercise: Resisted external rotation
Sport: Figure skating turn

Knee—sagittal
Flexion
Exercise: Leg (knee) curl
Sport: Diving tuck

Extension
Exercise: Leg (knee) extension
Sport: Volleyball block

Ankle—frontal
Inversion
Exercise: Resisted inversion
Sport: Football dribbling

Eversion
Exercise: Resisted eversion
Sport: Speed skating

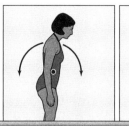
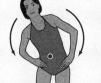

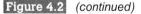
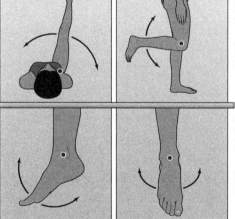

Figure 4.2 *(continued)*

Reprinted, by permission, E. Harman, 2008, Biomechanics of resistance exercise. In *Essentials of strength training and conditioning,* 3rd ed., by National Strength and Conditioning Association, edited by T.R. Baechle and R.W. Earle (Champaign, IL: Human Kinetics), 88-89. Adapted from E.A. Harman, M. Johnson, and P.N. Frykman 1992, "A movement-oriented approach to exercise prescription," *NSCA Journal* 14(1): 47-54.

action has important implications for enhancing the integrity of the knee joint during the squatting movement. The hamstring muscle group exerts a counter-regulatory pull on the tibia, helping to neutralise the anterior tibiofemoral shear imparted by the quadriceps and thus alleviating stress on the anterior cruciate ligament (Escamilla 2001). As a result, the hamstrings function both as hip extensor and knee flexor, and their length remains fairly constant throughout the movement, allowing for a relatively consistent force output throughout the squatting movement when the hip axis is above the knee axis (in relation to the horizontal plane). The rectus femoris in the quadriceps group is another bi-articular muscle, acting as both hip flexor and knee extensor during squatting. The rectus femoris shortens at one end while lengthening at the other end during the squat, with little if any net change in length throughout the movement (Schoenfeld 2010).

Safety and Risk of Injury in Resistance Training: Posture, Body Alignment and Range of Motion

Despite the relatively low risk of injury posed by resistance training, instructors should further minimise the likelihood of injury through appropriate risk management. The following section assesses the optimal recommended range of motion for performing exercises involving the main joints of the body, namely the shoulders, vertebral column and knees.

Shoulders

The shoulder is particularly prone to injury during resistance training, due to both its structure and the forces to which it is subjected during a training session. Similar to the hip, the shoulder is a multiplanar joint; as such it is capable of rotating in all directions. Whilst the hip is a stable ball-and-socket joint, the glenoid cavity of the shoulder, which holds the head of the humerus, is not a true socket. Therefore it is significantly less stable. It is maintained by a complex lattice-type network of connective tissues (figure 4.3).

The shoulder joint has the greatest range of motion of all the joints in the human body. The head of the humerus has the ability to move 2.5 centimetres out of the glenoid cavity during normal movement. This characteristic can also contribute to its vulnerability. The stability of the shoulder largely depends on the glenoid

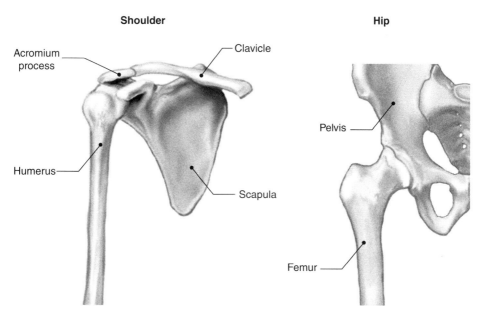

Shoulder

Acromium process

Clavicle

Humerus

Scapula

Hip

Pelvis

Femur

Figure 4.3 The shoulder joint has little bony support in contrast to the hip joint, which incorporates a deep and firm socket.

Harman 1994

labrum, the joint synovium and the capsules, ligaments, muscles, tendons and bursae that surround it (Pappas et al. 1983). Rotator cuff muscles (supraspinatus, infraspinatus, subscapularis and teres minor) and pectorals are particularly important in keeping the ball of the humerus in place. However, because of large possible ranges of motion of the shoulders, their various structures can easily impinge on one another, causing instability, tendinitis, inflammation and degeneration of contiguous tissue. Repetitive high forces generated during some resistance exercises, such as bench or shoulder presses, can result in tearing of ligaments, muscles and tendons (Harman 2008). Repetitive movement of abduction with external or internal rotation in the extreme range of motion may result in neural alteration (Colado and Garcia-Masso 2009). Examples of humeral-abducted and external-rotated exercises are the lateral pull-down, shoulder press behind the neck and supine pull-over with extensive ranges of motion. In order to avoid extreme risk positions participants should perform this exercise in front of the face for the lateral pull-down and vertical shoulder press and with the arm held at a 30-degree angle, forward with respect to the scapular plane (Colado and Garcia-Masso 2009). Exercises that use the extreme humeral abducted and internal rotated positions include the lateral arm raise with extreme internal rotation and upright row. These exercises can be a good option for strengthening the middle deltoid and supraspinatus; however, performing an excessive volume of repetitions with an internal rotation of the glenohumeral joint throughout large range of motion (>80 degrees or lifting the arm above shoulder level) can lead to rotator cuff impingement (figure 4.4) (Durall et al. 2001).

In addition, repetitive and heavy loaded movements of glenohumeral extreme horizontal abduction in individuals with a short training history can generate instability in the anterior region of the

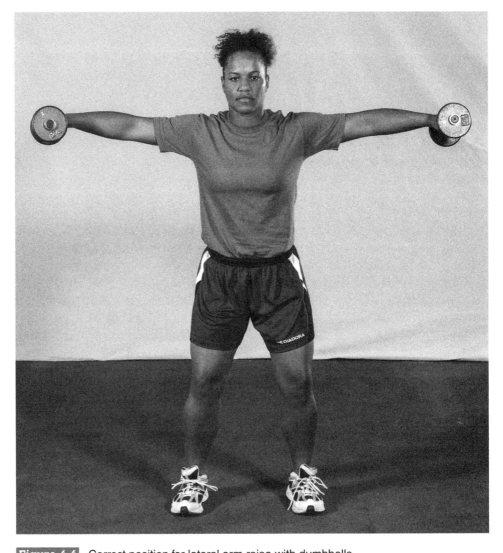

Figure 4.4   Correct position for lateral arm raise with dumbbells.

Reprinted from NSCA, 2008, *Essentials of strength training and conditioning,* 3rd ed. (Champaign, IL: Human Kinetics).

shoulders. Thus it is recommended that participants avoid or reduce high volumes of exercises such as bench press with a flat grip or dumbbell flys performed through a large range of motion. Excessive horizontal abduction during the bench press can be avoided by limiting hand spacing to 1.5 times the shoulder width, placing a cushion or roll on the chest or using a range of motion (ROM) limiting stop on a machine or self-spotting rack. Likewise, limiting hand spacing and horizontal abduction on a chest press machine protects the anterior glenohumeral capsuloligamentous restraints (Durall et al. 2001). Another extreme movement to minimise during press-type exercises is excessive internal rotation when the arm reaches a 90-degree angle of shoulder flexion, as in push-ups or the shoulder bench press, where a large degree of internal rotation is usually performed at the end of the concentric phase (Colado and Garcia-Masso 2009).

For general fitness purposes, members of the general population doing strength and conditioning exercises should avoid prolonged or high-volume exercises that involve raising the arms at or above shoulder level (Colado and Garcia-Masso 2009).

Vertebral Column

In a standing position, any force exerted with the upper body must be transmitted through the back to the legs and ground. The spine is comprised of 24 mobile vertebral segments, each displaying 3 degrees of freedom. Individually and as a unit, the spine is capable of flexion and extension in the sagittal plane, lateral flexion in the frontal plane and rotation in the transverse plane. The vertebral segments display a tapered appearance from top to bottom, with the vertebral bodies becoming progressively larger and thicker from the cervical to lumbar regions. The spine is involved directly or indirectly in most lifts because any weight supported by the arms or shoulders transmits force to the back. When a weight is supported in the hands or on the shoulders and the trunk is inclined forward, there is great torque around the lower intervertebral discs due to the large horizontal distance between the lower back and the weight. The back muscles operate at an extremely low mechanical advantage because the perpendicular distance from the line of action of the spinal erector muscles to the intervertebral discs is much shorter (about 5 centimetres) than the horizontal distance from the weight to the discs. As a result, the muscles must exert forces that frequently exceed 10 times the weight lifted. These forces act to squeeze the intervertebral discs between the adjacent vertebral bodies and can lead to possible injury or degenerative process. Figure 4.5 shows a hypothetical example of the compressive force (kilopascals) acting

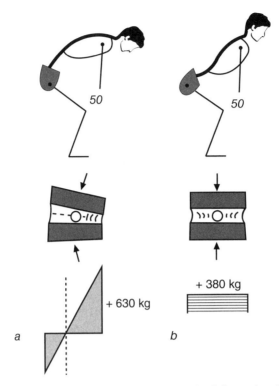

Figure 4.5 Compression load on the lumbar intervertebral discs when lifting a 50-kilogram weight with *(a)* incorrect or *(b)* correct techniques.

Reprinted, by permission, from Zatsiorsky, 2006, *Science and practice of strength training*, 2nd ed. (Champaign, IL: Human Kinetics), 148.

on lumbar intervertebral discs when lifting a 50-kilogram load with an incorrect (flexed back) or correct (neutral back) technique (Zatsiorsky and Kraemer 2006). A normal, slightly arched (lordotic) back has been found to be superior to a rounded back for avoiding injury to vertebrae, discs, facet joints, ligaments and muscles of the back. In addition, the lower-back muscles are capable of exerting considerably higher forces when the back forms a neutral position rather than flexed pattern (Harman 2008).

A fundamental guideline for resistance exercise practitioners is to maintain the spine in a neutral position, which is an intermediate position between maximum flexion and extension that respects the normal curvature of the vertebral column (Colado and Garcia-Masso 2009). The vertebral column is naturally S-shaped, being slightly rounded (kyphotic) in the thoracic spine and lordotic in the lumbar spine. The spine can support a greater axial load by maintaining the correct position of physiological curvatures. Any situation that alters the normal curvatures can increase the risk of acute injury or, if repeated many times, of degenerative injury. For instance, maintaining a seated position for long periods of time is not advisable. In addition it is better to perform exercises that move weight vertically from a standing position than to maintain a vertical seated position, which can lead to an inversion of the spine's curvature (Colado and Garcia-Masso 2009). Performing exercises from a standing position, such as a biceps curl or lateral arm rise, demand an activation of trunk musculature and stabilisation of the vertebral column in order to maintain a correct spinal position. Such a position can be demanding on participants with little training background or reduced functional musculature in the trunk. Here, in order to progress, the use of an inclined bench (at a 110- to 115-degree angle) can assist in the early stages of training.

For flexion–extension movements that occur while standing, such as the squat or overhead shoulder press or jerk, it is also important to maintain spinal integrity by contracting the diaphragm and deep muscles of the torso in order to stabilise the trunk. Because the abdomen is mainly composed of fluid and usually contains very little gas, it is virtually incompressible. When the surrounding abdominal and lumbar muscles contract, they will produce a very strong, supportive fluid ball that stabilises and protects the spine (figure 4.6).

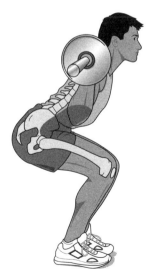

Figure 4.6 Fluid ball resulting from contraction of the trunk muscles.

Reprinted, by permission, E. Harman, 2008, Biomechanics of resistance exercise. In *Essentials of strength training and conditioning,* 3rd ed., by National Strength Training and Conditioning Association, edited by T.R. Baechle and R.W. Earle (Champaign, IL: Human Kinetics), 85.

When performing squatting exercises such as the back squat, the spine can very vulnerable. During both the ascent and descent phases, the lumbar spine is better able to handle compressive force than shearing force. Participants should maintain a normal lordotic curve, where the natural curve of the lumbar spine is evident, and should hold the vertebral column rigid throughout the movement, through a neutral position with additional thoracic extension (Schoenfeld 2010). Correct vertebral alignment is facilitated by maintaining the eyeline straight ahead or slightly upward. This reduces the tendency for unwanted flexion, predominantly in the thoracic region (Donnelly, Berg, and Fiske 2006). Although some forward lean is sometimes necessary to maintain stability, especially when performing deep squats, athletes should attempt to keep the trunk as upright as possible to minimise shear and to maintain the line of action within the base of support. No lateral movement should take place at any time (Schoenfeld 2010).

As a general recommendation, participants should perform standing resistance training exercises with the lower back maintaining evidence of the lumbar curve throughout all movements (Harman 2008).

Knees

The knee is one of the most complex joints in the body. As a result of its location between two long levers (the upper and lower leg), participants should pay considerable attention when performing lower-body exercises such as the squat, lunges or jumping actions. Flexion and extension around the knee occur almost exclusively in the sagittal plane. Rotation in the frontal plane and transverse plane is prevented mainly by stabilising ligamentous and cartilaginous structures. Fortunately, in training, resistive torques occur almost exclusively within the knee's normal plane of rotation. Of the various components of the knee, the patella and surrounding tissue are most susceptible to the kinds of forces encountered in resistance training (Colado and Garcia-Masso 2009). The patella's main function is to hold the quadriceps tendon away from the knee's axis of rotation, thereby increasing the moment arm of the quadriceps group and its mechanical advantage (see figure 4.7) (Harman 2008).

It has been postulated that the repetitive high force acting on the patellar tendon during some resistance training exercises such as the squat can damage knee ligaments and tendon structures and induce knee instability (Shoemaker and Markolf 1985; Yack, Collins, and Whiedon 1993; Klein 1961). However, further studies concluded that the full and parallel squats did not increase joint laxity or insta-

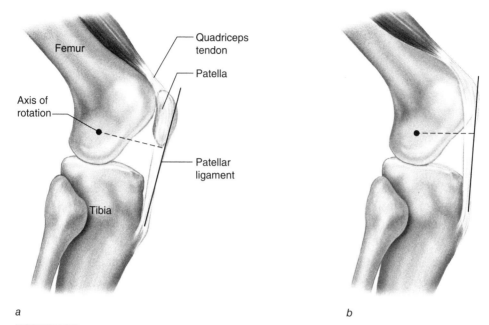

a   *b*

Figure 4.7 *(a)* The patella improves the moment arm by maintaining the quadriceps tendon's distance from the knee's axis of rotation; *(b)* the absence of the patella shortens the moment arm through which the muscle force acts, thereby reducing the muscle's mechanical advantage.

bility. When completing these movements or similar exercises such as lunges with appropriate preparation and technique, there is no reason for contraindicated outcomes to occur (Neitzel and Davies 2000; Schoenfeld 2010). Inappropriate athletic conditioning and excessive training volume have been associated with fatigue and loss of motor control during squatting exercises. In such cases a change in the movement of the patella, such as excessive internal or external rotation of the lower extremities during the descent and ascent phases, can damage the joint structure (Schoenfeld 2010).

Previously instructors have been cautioned against prescribing the deep squat in their resistance training programmes; critics cite an increased potential for injury to soft tissue in the knee during a high degree of flexion (Kellis et al. 2005). These concerns, however, appear largely unwarranted (Schoenfeld 2010). Although it is true that shear forces tend to increase with deeper knee angles, forces on the anterior and posterior cruciate ligaments actually decrease at high flexion. As a result of compressive force peaking at high degrees of knee flexion, the greatest risk of injury during deep squatting would appear to be on menisci and joint cartilage, which are placed under increased stress at high flexion angles (Li et al. 2004; Escamilla 2001). Unfortunately, no guidelines currently exist for determining at what magnitude of force injury may occur. The knee may be susceptible to patellofemoral degeneration, given the high amount of patellofemoral stress that arises from the contact of the underside of the patella with the articulating aspect of the femur during high flexion (Escamilla 2001). This can lead to disorders such as chondromalacia, osteoarthritis and osteochondritis. It is therefore essential to consider participants' special level of conditioning, anthropometric relationship or their eventual pathologic condition when determining optimal squat depth. Conversely, connective tissue adapts to regimented resistance training by increasing its tolerance level, which further reduces the prospect of injury under loaded conditions (Buchanan and Marsh 2002). In assessing the sport-specific demands of an individual and the need to regularly perform the full-depth squat exercise, instructors should counsel participants to maintain good technique and to avoid bouncing and loss of motor control during the full squat; this can result in beneficial outcomes such as increased stability and tolerance to loads (Schoenfeld 2010).

For general fitness purposes, when training novice practitioners or athletes without special requirements to perform the full squat, instructors should limit the knee flexion to 90 degrees (Colado and Garcia-Masso 2009) or 100 degrees (parallel squat) (Escamilla 2001) and give special attention to controlling excessive internal and external rotation of the tibia and hyperextension of the knee before allowing participants to progress to the full depth.

Even if there is no confirmed evidence by which an exercise provides a contraindication per se, instructors have to be confident that the individuals they are working with are able to perform all the selected strength and conditioning exercises with good technique and motor control throughout the entire training session, or the risk of injury will be increased.

Safe and Effective Spotting Techniques

For resistance training to be safe and effective, all participants and instructors in a facility should follow safety rules. The following safety and etiquette checklist is advised to ensure an optimal resistance training environment (Ratamess 2012a).

- Obtain medical clearance before beginning training. According to their joint position statement, the American Heart Association (AHA) and the American College of Sports Medicine (ACSM) recommend that all individuals be screened prior to participation with a medical history questionnaire or health appraisal document (AHA/ ACSM 1998).

■ Experienced instructors should screen the clients they work with on a regular basis in order to determine their strengths and weaknesses related to motor performance. For instance, many athletes with little experience in resistance training usually demonstrate a limited range of movement at the hip and ankle that can impede them from performing the correct body shapes, positions and movements during the squatting technique. In such instances, novice athletes can start with other exercises such as the leg press or use a squat with a decreased load and limited range of motion combined with flexibility exercises aimed to improve motor performance before progressing to higher loads and more intense squat training.

■ Participants should wear appropriate clothing and sports shoes (stable and comfortable) in order to allow for optimal range of motion. Clothing should reflect ambient temperature in order to permit participants to maintain a comfortable body temperature in various conditions (Ratamess 2012a).

■ Both the instructor and the client must know the correct procedures for using each training device (e.g., machines, bands or free weights); prior checks of the correct movement and pieces as well as the appropriate functions must be completed for equipment with every use. Each machine should have an adjustment point; for example, in performing a leg extension exercise, the knee should be aligned with the machine's axis of rotation, and the seat or back support should adjust to permit the user to use it effectively. When using the chest press machine, the seat should allow the user to set the grip height or position at the lower (sternal) chest level. If this is not possible, the risk of injury or accidents may increase (Faigenbaum et al. 2011).

■ No clients will be permitted to complete resistance training exercises until they are able to demonstrate correct technique. Incorrect technique, especially with free-weight exercises, can increase the risk of injury or accidents (Faigenbaum et al. 2011).

■ Do not bounce the weight stack or place fingers near the stack when someone is using it.

■ Do not disturb participants while they are in the middle of completing a set. Distraction can place the weightlifter at higher risk for injury or can result in poor performance of the exercise.

■ Never attempt to lift excessive loads, continuously complete repetitions to failure or complete forced repetitions without a spotter.

The safety rack should always be in position. For certain exercises, such as squat, bench press and its variations or the shoulder press, one, two or even three spotters, depending on the amount of the weight, are recommended.

- Control dumbbells and clamps to prevent the weight from slipping. Secure clamps or collars prevent plates from slipping off one or both sides, perhaps striking the lifter and causing injury.

- Be careful when loading and unloading bars, making sure that bars are equally loaded on both ends.

- Especially when using free weights, make sure the lifter has sufficient space for completing the movements required. Lifting too close to other practitioners may result in increased chances of injury through contact with resistance equipment. This is a very important consideration when clients are performing Olympic lifts. Standards have been set by several organisations such as the NSCA that detail appropriate space between pieces of weightlifting equipment (Greenwood and Greenwood 2008).

- Be sure that participants are always in an appropriately stable position when beginning resistance exercises.

- Weights should be lifted and replaced in a controlled manner (speeds can vary, but lifters should always exhibit control). Correct loading is essential to assisting in controlling weights, especially during the eccentric phase. Beginners usually do not adequately control the eccentric phase; therefore they are more likely to suffer injury due to uncontrolled actions. In some cases, such as after completing weightlifting exercises, clients drop or throw free weights on the platform because it is easier than lowering the weight in a controlled, sequential manner back to the floor.

- In order to reduce the risk of related lower-back injuries when lifting weights from the floor, emphasise lower-body actions and neutral back posture to maintain spinal integrity and stability while minimising spinal loading. Lumbar extensor muscles contract to increase spine rigidity. This maintains the lordotic arch, which reduces spinal shear stress. This important weightlifting technique should ideally be learned before adolescence (Faigenbaum and Myer 2012). It could be described as retracting the shoulder girdle, sticking the chest out and bracing the core. This position should be maintained for all resistance exercises, not solely for lifting weights off the ground (Ratamess 2012a).

- It is important to complete and understand the correct breathing patterns during the lift, since this assists greatly in stabilising the body and maintaining spinal integrity, and it reduces both the risk of injury and cardiovascular stress. In general, appropriate breathing technique—exhaling on the positive or concentric phase and inhaling on the negative or eccentric phase—should be performed to maximise performance and reduce cardiovascular stress. However there are some exceptions, such as when training with heavy or maximal loads (>85 percent 1RM) or performing movements that require a maximal explosive effort. In this situation, holding one's breath (Valsalva manoeuvre) increases intra-abdominal, intrathoracic pressure and torso rigidity. For example, weightlifters may inhale prior to engaging with the lift from the floor in a clean and jerk, holding their breath to maintain spinal integrity throughout the whole of the movement until they have caught the bar and managed to stand erect with the bar across the shoulders in preparation for completing the jerk. In order to move maximal or near-maximal loads during weightlifting or similar activities, holding the breath to stabilise the spine allows clients to overcome the striking region that is the weakest part of the exercise, where the vulnerability of the lower back increases. It is important to point out that examples of high strength and power during training and competition are the exception to the breathing principle, and the general principles previously are advocated in the majority of circumstances (Ratamess 2012a).

Spotting Free-Weight Exercises

A spotter is someone who assists lifters with the execution of an exercise in order to help them complete it. The spotter's primary responsibility is to protect the lifter from possible injuries (Earle and Baechle 2008).

Whilst it may appear obvious, spotters must be familiar with exercises that they are about to assist with. Failure to do this may increase the risk of injury to both the lifter and the spotter.

Free-weight exercises performed over the head (e.g., barbell shoulder press or push jerk), with the bar on the back (e.g., back squat), racked interiorly on the shoulders (e.g., front squat) or over the face (e.g., lying triceps extension) are more challenging for participants to correctly execute than those in which the bar or dumbbells are held or raised at the sides or in front of the body (e.g., lateral shoulder raise or barbell biceps curl, respectively). Therefore, these exercises should demand appropriate technique and control, as well as spotter assistance, when the load is close to maximal (>80 percent 1RM) or the number of repetitions per set approaches failure. Overhead exercises, ones with the bar held on the back or front shoulders, and over-the-face exercises (especially using dumbbells) require considerably more skill on the part of the spotter; these have the potential to be the most dangerous. Spotting dumbbell exercises typically requires more skill than spotting barbell exercises because there are two pieces of equipment that can move independently to observe and spot.

Weightlifting exercises (or their associated derivatives) should not be spotted. In this case, instructors should teach participants to release the bar to the front and move backwards or to allow the increased angular backward momentum to continue and then jump forward if any of these conditions occur. For these reasons, the surrounding area or platform should be cleared of other practitioners and equipment before such exercises are performed (Earle and Baechle 2008).

With the exception of the Smith machine, machine exercises usually do not require spotters unless the programme requires forced repetitions, but this would be most appropriate for experienced participants with an advanced training history. With novice practitioners the instructor's main function is to assist the participants in adequate execution of the movement, emphasising the complete range of motion and the correct use of the device.

Spotting Overhead Exercises and Those With the Bar on the Back or Front Shoulders

Ideally this type of exercise should be performed inside a power rack with the safety bars secured in place at an appropriate height, based on the lifter's somatotype, and range of movement to be used within the repetitions. The principal spotter should stand behind the lifter and the assistant spotters should stand on the sides (one on the left and the other on the right). Out-of-the-rack exercises (e.g., forward step lunge or step-up) with heavy weights should only be completed by well-trained and skilled athletes and spotted by experienced fitness professionals (Earle and Baechle 2008). When only one spotter spots for a squat, he or she should be positioned behind the lifter, and should follow the movement down and up in each repetition to help the lifter maintain proper position. Spotters should avoid pushing the athlete forward when assisting. If support is required, the spotters will lift their arms up so that the crease of their elbows and upper arms drive support under the lifter's armpits. Spotters must help the lifter maintain the correct posture of the lumbar spine and vertebral column, as described previously, and support the lifter as if they were completing the squat themselves, that is, driving up with the legs and retaining postural integrity throughout.

Spotting Over-the-Face Exercises

When spotting over-the-face barbell exercises, the spotter must grasp the bar with an alternated grip, usually inside the lifter's grip (figure 4.8).

Because the movement of the bar can follow a curved trajectory, in some exercises (e.g. lying triceps extension, barbell pull-over), the spotter will use an alternated grip to pick up the bar and return it to the floor but a supinated grip to spot the bar. This helps ensure

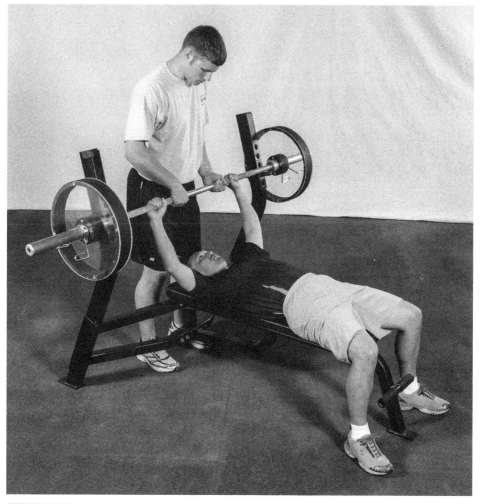

Figure 4.8 Recommended grip position for spotter during over-the-face exercise.

that the bar does not roll out of the spotter's hands and onto the athlete's face or neck during assistance.

Spotting Dumbbell Exercises

For dumbbell exercises, it is important to spot as close to the dumbbells as possible or, in a number of exercises, to spot the dumbbell itself or to grasp the wrist. Although some people advocate spotting dumbbell movements by placing the hands on the lifter's upper arms or elbows (figure 4.9a), this procedure is not recommended because it increases the risk of injury if the lifter is not able to control the weight and suddenly externally rotates the arm and loses the control of the weight. If this happens, the spotter will not be in a position to stop the dumbbells. Spotting at the forearms near the wrists (figure 4.9b) provides a safer technique. Note that for some exercises (e.g., dumbbell pull-over and overhead dumbbell triceps extension), the spotter must place hands on the dumbbell itself.

Number of Spotters

The number of spotters needed is largely determined by the exercise, the load being lifted and the experience, ability and strength level of the lifters and spotters. Once the load exceeds the spotter's ability to effectively assist the lifter, an additional spotter must become involved. When two or three spotters are needed, they must coordinate their actions with those of the lifter.

Prior to beginning a set, the spotters should discuss with the lifters what method will be used to support them, the amount of assistance they should provide and whether a lift-off (refers to moving the bar from the upright supports to a position from which the lifter can begin the exercise) and assistance to rack the weight after completion of the exercise are needed. They should reach an agreement about when the spotters will intervene and assist, as well as confirm what contact may be made during spotting, how many repetitions the lifter is planning on completing and the potential for arriving to failure or doing forced repetitions. In addition, the spotters should not crowd the lifters; they must give them adequate space to complete the exercise. Although this seems like a lot of information, effective communication and the relationship between the spotter and the lifter are crucial to a safe and effective outcome.

Experienced spotters must know and feel when they should provide the required assistance in order to apply sufficient force to keep the resistance moving, but they should not take away from the lifter's effort. This ensures that the lifter works maximally but receives appropriate support to successfully complete a repetition. In general,

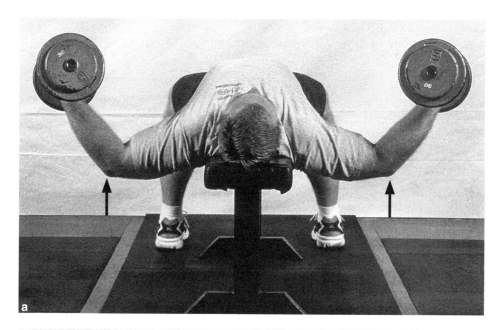

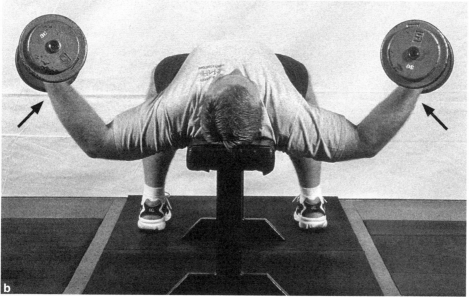

Figure 4.9 *(a)* Incorrect and *(b)* correct dumbbell spotting location.

the spotter should not take the bar or resistance away completely unless required to do so for safety reasons, or during a testing procedure. If the lifter cannot contribute anything to the completion of the repetition, the spotter should take the bar (if possible) quickly and smoothly, trying to avoid abrupt changes in the amount of load being handled by the lifter. The lifter should try to stay with the bar until it is racked or returned to the starting position. This helps protect both the spotter and lifter from accidents and possible injuries. They should both stay focused and avoid becoming distracted by others in the gym.

Use of Lifting Belts

Although research is inconclusive about whether the use of a lifting belt either effectively lowers the rate of injury or has no effect (Renfro and Ebben 2006), its uses may be appropriate depending on the type of exercise performed and the relative weight being lifted. A lifting belt can be worn for exercises that place stress on the lower back and during sets that use near-maximal or maximal loads (>80 percent 1RM) (Lander et al. 1992). Using such a belt may improve the capability of the lifter to stabilise the spine during lifting by helping to increase intra-abdominal pressure (IAP) and decrease the compressive force on the lumbar discs. Lifting belts can assist the spinal erector muscles in supporting the spine. The application of additional compressive force in this region will help reduce any excessive compressive loading on the spinal discs at the same time (Faigenbaum and Liatsos 1994). Furthermore lifting belts can keep the back from arching excessively in the lumbar spine during overhead lifting. Participants receive a greater sense of support when wearing a lifting belt (Faigenbaum and Liatsos 1994). A significant drawback to using a lifting belt is that it may reduce opportunities for training the abdominal and lower-back muscles. Furthermore, no lifting belt is needed for exercises that do not stress the lower back, or for exercises that do stress the lower back (e.g., back squat or dead lift) but involve the use of light loads (<80 percent 1RM) (Earle and Baechle 2008). Lifting belts may be even more useful when participants plan to do maximal sets to failure or forced repetitions with submaximal loads. During this type of training, fatigue might affect the proper exercise execution and create additional strain on the lower spine (Lander et al. 1992).

In summary, although wearing a lifting belt may not promote an increase in the total applied force, it seems that it can induce some positive effects for resistance training practitioners: reduce spinal compression, stabilise the spine, increase motor unit recruitment in prime movers, and possibly increase resistance exercise velocity (Renfro and Ebben 2006). In order to avoid detrimental weakening effects due to overuse of lifting belts, lifters should wear them only when mobilising heavy or maximal weight as well as when doing sets to failure or forced repetitions, but they should not wear belts when training with lighter loads, during warm-ups or even during the rest period in between heavy resistance training workouts. Furthermore, practitioners should not become too dependent on the support of the lifting belts. In fact, lifters who routinely wear a belt for every set should be extremely strong when lifting without belt.

Warming Up for Resistance Training

The warm-up is an essential introductory part of the training session that helps participants prepare both mentally and physically for the training session (Siff 2004; Jeffreys 2008). Warm-up techniques can be broadly classified into two major categories: passive warm-ups and active warm-ups. Passive warm-ups involve raising the muscle temperature or core temperature by some external means. Various methods include hot showers or baths, saunas, diathermy and heating pads. Passive heating increases both muscle and core temperature without depleting energy substrates (Bishop 2003a). Meanwhile, active warm-ups involve exercise. They are likely to induce greater metabolic and cardiovascular changes than passive warm-up procedures, and they also potentially disrupt transient connective tissue bonds and improve the body's neuromuscular preparedness for the specific task ahead (Jeffreys 2008; Bishop 2003a).

A typical active warm-up for resistance training should involve two phases: general and specific. The purpose of a general warm-up is to increase the functional potential of the body as a whole, whereas

 Examples of a Typical Lower-Body Resistance Training Warm-Up Involving Both General and Specific Phases

General warm-up
- Five minutes of low-intensity aerobic exercises: jogging and three low-intensity stretching exercises (one leg rise for hamstring, forward lunge and seated toe touch).

Specific warm-up
- Medicine ball twist 1 × 20
- Medicine ball wood chops 1 × 10
- Straddled toe touch 2 × 5
- Dynamic quadriceps stretch 1 × 5
- Medicine ball squat 1 × 5 to 8
- Back squat using 50 percent of the load to be used during the main part of workout

the goal of the specific phase is to establish the optimal relationship between warm-up and the forthcoming resistance exercises (Siff 2004). A typical general warm-up can last 5 to 10 minutes (Ratamess 2012b). This first phase usually begins with light-intensity exercises such as jogging, cycling or easy stretching or active displacements. The intensity is increased progressively in order to lead participants towards the specific phase, which is aimed to optimise their preparation for the main part of the workout. However, for resistance exercises, a general warm-up does not always involve aerobic exercise such as cycling or jogging. Global callisthenic movements, easy stretching and dynamic flexibility movements are also appropriate.

A specific warm-up phase can last 8 to 12 minutes (Jeffreys 2008). Its structure varies greatly depending on the sport or activity. For resistance training, the specific part of the warm-up can involve several (four to six) dynamic exercises, which can be completed using bands or a medicine ball as required. Before commencing the main part of the workout, participants should perform one or two sets of a few repetitions (four to eight) with a light to moderate load of the principal multijoint exercise to be trained (Ratamess 2012b). It appears that a specific warm-up can provide further benefits in addition to those provided by a general, active warm-up, possibly by optimising the required neuromuscular activation for the main part of the workout (Bishop 2003b). The following list depicts examples of general and specific warm-ups for lower-body resistance training.

Effects of the Warm-Up

The following list depicts the ways in which a proper warm-up positively affects performance (Bishop 2003a):

Temperature related

- Decreases resistance of muscles and joints
- Increases release of oxygen from haemoglobin and myoglobin
- Speeds up metabolic reactions
- Increases nerve conduction rate
- Increases thermoregulatory strain

Non-temperature related

- Increases blood flow to muscles
- Raises baseline oxygen consumption
- Enhances postactivation potentiation
- Psychologically prepares participant for main routine

The warm-up movements should speed up contraction and relaxation of both agonist and antagonist muscles, which improves strength, power, rate of force development and reaction time (Jeffreys 2008). Whilst the influence of warming up on injury prevention is still unclear (Bishop 2003a), some studies suggest that it prevents muscular or connective tissue injury (Olsen et al. 2004; Olsen et al. 2005). At the very least, a structured warm-up can enhance performance and may reduce injury potential (Ratamess 2012b). Currently no evidence suggests that a warm-up is detrimental to performance. Some evidence suggests that under certain circumstances, a low-volume and high-intensity resistance training exercise (>80 percent 1RM) warm-up increases neuromuscular activation and therefore increases the performance in explosive actions performed next (Tillin and Bishop 2009). It has also been hypothesised that warming up may have a number of psychological effects (Bishop 2003a).

Dynamic Versus Static Flexibility Exercise

For many years, static stretching exercises were widely accepted for use in warm-ups with the intent to reduce injury and increase the range of motion as well as performance. However, during the last 20 years, researchers have yielded some interesting findings regarding the possible negative effects as well as the possible increase of muscular injury risk with intense (not light) stretching prior to strength and power events (Stone et al. 2006; Heiderscheit et al. 2010). Muscle strength, power and speed performance (e.g., vertical jump height, power, agility and sprint speed) may be reduced (by up to 30 percent) immediately following or during the first 2 hours after doing intense or long-duration static stretching exercise warm-up protocols compared to a general warm-up that does not include stretching (Andersen 2005; Stone et al. 2006; Young 2007; Ratamess 2012b). Conversely, dynamic flexibility exercises such as large-limb amplitude movements that involve exaggerated lunges or arm rotations have not elicited any detrimental effects on explosive efforts, speed or strength performance; in contrast, they have positively influenced these types of activities (Thacker et al. 2004). The possible negative effects of static stretching have been associated with the intensity and duration of the exercise, particularly holding extreme positions for more than 30 seconds (Young 2007). Holding stretches for more than 45 seconds (Kay and Blazevich 2012) has been associated with significant decreases in power and speed performance. Therefore the use of light-intensity stretching protocols (small range of motion) of short duration (5 to 10 seconds per repetition) (Young 2007), or in positions held for less than 30 seconds (Kay and Blazevich 2012), combined with dynamic flexibility exercises has been proposed as an optimal alternative for increasing performance (Ratamess 2012b; McHugh and Cosgrave 2010).

Training Status and Individual Differences in Resistance Training Practitioners

According to the experience, performance and type of specific sports, training status of resistance trained individuals can fall along a continuum that ranges from beginners to high-performance athletes. However, genetic endowment or prior motor experiences outside of resistance training often make it difficult to classify the level of some participants on this continuum. Notwithstanding, for the purposes of this chapter, a beginner has no or very little experience in resistance training and has a large potential window of adaptation available. An intermediate-trained participant has had a minimum of four months of regularly progressive resistance training and has attained significant and measurable increases in strength; for instance, a male participant who has a 1RM of 1 kilogram per kilograms of body weight (BW) in the bench press or more than 1.2 kilogram per kilograms BW in the back squat (Naclerio 2009). An advanced participant has spent at least one year following a regularly progressive resistance training programme and has experienced a substantial level of adaptation; for instance, a male participant who has an 1RM of >1.25 kilogram per kilograms BW in bench press or >1.5 kilogram per kilograms BW in back squat (Naclerio 2009).

Training status identification helps instructors better analyse the rate and magnitude of progression. Novice participants will respond favourably to any programme, thereby making it difficult for instructors to evaluate the real effectiveness of the programme at the initial stage. However, as their level of performance increases, their rate of progression will begin to decrease, and instructors will need to apply more specific, well-designed resistance training programmes (ACSM 2002). In general, the expected maximum strength increase over a training period that ranges from four weeks to two years is approximately 40 percent for novices, 20 percent for intermediate participants, 16 percent for those with recreational training, 10 percent in recreational yet advanced resistance-trained practitioners and only 2 percent for elite resistance-trained athletes (ACSM 2002).

As a general recommendation, the initial phase of the resistance training programme should be characterised by low-intensity or low-volume training where enhanced technique and general conditioning are the primary goals; however, as participants progress and become more conditioned, they will require more effective and specific training methods in order to continue progressing (Ratamess 2012c).

Dose–Response Relationship for Different Resistance Training Goals

Historically, it has been difficult and controversial to determine the ideal dose of resistance training with an optimal relationship among volume, intensity and frequency associated with each special goal (strength, power, muscle endurance or hypertrophy).

Meta-analysis researchers have demonstrated that for novice individuals, maximal strength gains are elicited using 60 percent of 1RM, three days per week, with a training volume of three or four sets per muscle group. Recreationally intermediate resistance-trained practitioners exhibit maximal strength gains with a mean training intensity of 80 percent of 1RM, two days per week, and a mean volume of four sets. For the well-trained athlete, maximal strength gains are elicited from training at 85 percent of 1RM, two days per week, and with a mean training volume of eight sets per muscle group (Peterson et al. 2005).

Of the various prescription variables of resistance training, volume has undoubtedly received the most research attention. Performing a single set of exercises per muscle group resulted in significant strength gains (Krieger 2009) and hypertrophy outcomes (Krieger 2010), particularly in novice or intermediate resistance-trained practitioners; this can be enough to maintain the level of strength in advanced athletes as well (Naclerio et al. 2011). However, using multiple sets is a superior approach for gaining strength in both novice and advanced athletes (Krieger 2010, Peterson et al. 2005). Specifically, performing two or three sets per exercise was associated with 46 percent greater strength gains than one set, and no significant additional benefit was observed for more than three sets (Krieger 2009). These findings applied to both trained and novice practitioners who practised both upper- and lower-body exercises at a variety of training frequencies. Even when training with four to six sets, participants have elicited more strength gains (around 13 percent) with two or three sets per exercise. It appears from a research perspective that there is a plateau in strength gains when training with more than three sets per exercise (Krieger 2009). It is important to highlight that the 13 percent increase in strength gains, even from a research perspective, failed to provide statistical significance; this impact on performance could contribute greatly to gains for high-performance athletes, but it is unlikely to transfer to other participants, and it is even less likely to be formally researched.

Unless adequately designed, overprescribing training variables initially accelerates strength gains, but subsequently causes the participant to plateau, decreasing muscular strength and causing adverse side effects associated with overreaching or overtraining (Halson and Jeukendrup 2004). In contrast, underprescribing training may be appropriately regarded as inefficient training. Thus, underprescription is less detrimental for most nonathletes than for advanced or competitive athletes, who will experience far greater consequences if their performances are hindered (Peterson et al. 2005).

An optimal dose–response relationship for maximal strength adaptation exists. The trends demonstrate that progressing training volume to reach eight sets of training per muscle group increases maximal strength in resistance exercises. For a particular exercise, the first set of training is responsible for close to 50 percent of overall net potential strength gain for both novice and trained participants, the latter of which will need three or four sets to achieve maximal effect for improving 1RM (Krieger 2009).

Clearly, both athletes and nonathletes require multiple sets of strength training for optimal muscular strength development per unit of time. Low-volume and single-set protocols drastically restrict the potential strength adaptation of athletes and nonathletes, respectively (Krieger 2009; Krieger 2010; Peterson et al. 2005; Ratamess 2012c).

Instructors should design training programmes for athletes by systematically setting goals. They must establish the primary objectives in order to maximise training effect per unit of time. Multiple goals can be achieved with an integrative approach that permits participants to express their maximum level of performance during competition. Table 4.1 depicts the number of sets per muscle group that should be performed over the entire resistance training session to meet the three main objectives (recover, increase or maintain strength) most commonly presented (Naclerio et al. 2011).

Table 4.1 Resistance Training: Optimal Training Volume and Goals for Athletes

Period	Starting	Pre-season	In-season
Goals	Recover strength	Increase strength	Maintain strength
Sets per muscle group per exercise	3 to 6 1 to 2	4 to 6 to 8 2 to 3 to 4	1 to 3 1
Total sets per session	8 to 15	24 to 27	6 to 10

Conclusion

With adequate supervision and appropriate technique, resistance training is safe and beneficial for improving performance and health regardless of age and level of conditioning. A qualified strength and conditioning instructor should always design the most appropriate resistance training programme for each individual participant, considering their specific goals for health or athletic performance. Knowledge of how different dose-responses (including intensity, volume and frequency) affect resistance training outcomes, as well as how different types of exercise provide specific patterns of resistance in the body, can help instructors develop safe and effective programmes to suit the specific needs of participants who engage in resistance training to enhance their physical performance, health, sense of well-being and self-confidence.

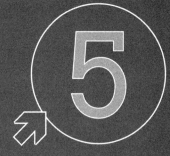

Safe Progressive Exercise Planning

Oscar Carballo Iglesias

Eliseo Iglesias-Soler

This chapter covers the aspects of prescribing safe exercises. The first portion of the chapter teaches instructors how to analyse participants' characteristics in order to adapt the doses and loads of exercises and routines to the capacities of each individual. The next section shows instructors how to adapt their communication in order to be well understood by their clients. Finally the chapter explains the changes that take place in the human body after progressive exercise. It also describes the principles of training such as overload, specificity and individual responsiveness.

Assessing Clients and Modifying Exercise Programmes

The National Strength and Conditioning Association (NSCA) defines the scope of practice for instructors by characterising them as 'health/fitness professionals who use an individual approach to assess, motivate, educate, and train clients regarding their health and fitness needs. They design safe and effective exercise programs and provide the guidance to help clients achieve their personal goals. In addition, they respond appropriately in emergency situations and refer clients to health care professionals when necessary' (Earle and Baechle 2004, p. 147).

This definition contains three parts: assessment, programme design and reassessment. In the first phase, in order to optimise safety during exercise testing and participation, instructors should use a health appraisal process to screen participants for risk factors and symptoms of chronic cardiovascular, pulmonary, metabolic and orthopaedic diseases. Instructors must gather and assess pertinent information regarding participants' personal health, medical conditions and lifestyle (table 5.1). According to the NSCA (Baechle and Earle 2008) two instruments are commonly used: the PAR-Q (Physical Activity Readiness Questionnaire) and the AHA/ACSM Health/Fitness Preparticipation Screening Questionnaire.

These variables are very similar to those that the American Heart Association (AHA) and American College of Sports Medicine (ACSM) have recommended since 1998 in their Health/Fitness Preparticipation Screening Questionnaire (ACSM 2009).

After conducting the health appraisal, the instructor needs to gather more information about the client's current level of fitness and skills before developing a programme. When identifying and selecting appropriate tests, instructors should keep the following factors in mind:

- Health status and functional capacity
- Age
- Sex
- Pretraining status (trained or untrained population)

Table 5.1 Health Appraisal Variables

Coronary risk factors	■ Family history ■ Cigarette smoking ■ Hypertension ■ Hypercholesterolemia ■ Impaired fasting glucose ■ Obesity ■ Sedentary lifestyle
Diagnosed disease	■ Coronary artery and pulmonary disease ■ Metabolic disease ■ Orthopaedic conditions and disease ■ Medications
Lifestyle	■ Dietary intake and eating habits ■ Exercise and activity patterns ■ Stress management

Based on NSCA 2008.

On the basis of the results obtained during the diagnostic process, the instructor may recommend an unsupervised, supervised or medically supervised exercise programme.

Next instructors should consider programme design. All effective exercise programmes are based on general training principles: specificity, overload, progression (Earle and Baechle 2004) and variability, as well as any modifications necessary for individual clients (Howley and Thompson 2012). Fitness programmes must address the needs, interests and limitations of the group being served. Instructors must think about equipment, activities and pace when planning a class for participants at either end of the spectrum in terms of age, fitness level and skill.

At the end of the programme, instructors should conduct another assessment to see the extent to which participants have fulfilled their goals. In the reassessment phase, instructors should adapt or modify programmes as needed or allow clients to change their goals. This feedback may take place eight or more weeks after the programme begins. Depending on their goals, participants may require more or less time to reach completion.

Providing Proper Dose–Response Relationship for Individual Participants

In order to prescribe effective training programmes, instructors must first identify a quantifiable relationship between dose (exercise) and response (specific health or fitness adaptations). Some studies have demonstrated that different training volumes and intensities elicit different magnitudes of strength gains, but they have only hinted at a dose–response trend (Rhea et al. 2003).

Of the training variables, volume has received the most attention from researchers, possibly because it is easier to control than training intensity or periodisation. Currently certain processes help instructors learn the effects of variables, such as intensity, frequency and volume, on physical fitness.

Aerobic

Different reviews have found that the higher the exercise intensity, the greater the increase in aerobic fitness. In their review Swain and Franklin (2006) conclude that if the total energy expenditure of exercise is held constant, exercise performed at a vigorous intensity appears to convey greater cardio protective benefits than exercise of a moderate intensity. Several studies associate vigorous physical activities with a reduced risk of coronary heart disease, decrease in diastolic blood pressure and increase in $\dot{V}O_2$max.

The ACSM (Garber et al. 2011) recommends the following guidelines for aerobic exercise:

- **Frequency:** Adults should get ≥5 days per week of moderate exercise or ≥3 days per week of vigorous exercise, or a combination of moderate and vigorous exercise 3 to 5 days per week.

- **Intensity:** Moderate and vigorous intensity is recommended for most adults. Light- to moderate-intensity exercise may be beneficial for people with poor fitness levels.

- **Time:** Most adults should do purposeful moderate exercise for 30 to 60 minutes per day, 5 days per week (at least 150 minutes per week), vigorous exercise for 20 to 60 minutes per day, 3 days per week (at least 60 minutes per week), or a combination of moderate and vigorous exercise each day.

- **Volume:** A target volume of 500 to 1,000 METs per minute per week is recommended. A daily pedometer step count of at least 7,000 steps per day is beneficial. Clients hoping to improve their volume can begin by working to increase their step count by 2,000 steps per day.

Resistance

A meta-analysis of the effects of resistance exercise on strength increases identified differences between trained and untrained participants, but did not find the same differences between men and women (Rhea et al. 2003). Table 5.2 summarises recommendations for increasing strength with resistance exercise.

Table 5.2   Recommendations for Resistance Exercise for Untrained and Trained Populations (Rhea et al. 2003)

	Training recommendations for optimal strength increases
Untrained population (exercising for less than 1 yr)	Work out at 60% of 1RM (1-repetition maximum) 4 sets per muscle group 3 days per week
Trained population	Work out 80% of 1RM 4 sets per muscle group 2 days per week

Adapted from Rhea et al. 2003.

In another meta-analysis, Peterson, Rhea and Alvar (2005) demonstrate that maximal strength gains are elicited among athletes who train two days per week at 85 percent of 1RM (intensity) and perform eight sets for each muscle group (volume). Training at lower volumes (1 to 3 sets) and intensities (50 to 70 percent 1RM) elicited minimal strength improvements among athletes. In terms of the effects of training frequency, the study shows no great difference between training two or three days per week.

The ACSM (Garber et al. 2011) recommends the following guidelines for resistance exercise:

- **Frequency:** Train each major muscle group two or three days per week.

- **Repetitions:**
  - 8 to 12 repetitions are recommended to improve strength and power in most adults.
  - 10 to 15 repetitions are effective in improving strength in middle-aged and older people who are just starting to exercise.
  - 15 to 20 repetitions are recommended for improving muscular endurance. Two to four sets are recommended for most adults for improving strength and power.

- **Sets:** A single set of resistance exercises can be effective, especially among older and novice exercisers.
  - 2 to 4 sets are recommended for improving strength and power for most adults.
  - At least two sets are effective for improving muscular endurance.

Flexibility and Neuromuscular Exercises

Flexibility training and neuromuscular exercise are also important components to consider when creating an exercise plan. The ACSM (Garber et al. 2011) recommends the following guidelines for improving flexibility:

- **Frequency:** At least two days per week are effective for improving joint range of motion, with the greatest gains occurring with daily exercise.

- **Intensity:** Participants should stretch to the point of feeling tightness or slight discomfort.

- **Time:** Most adults should hold a static stretch for 10 to 30 seconds. Older people may benefit from stretching longer (30 to 60 seconds). For PNF (proprioceptive neuromuscular facilitation) stretching, a 3- to 6-second contraction at 20 to 75 percent of maximum voluntary contraction, followed by a 10- to 30-second assisted stretch, is desirable.
- **Type:** A series of flexibility exercises for each of the major muscle–tendon units is recommended.

The ACSM (Garber et al., 2011) recommends the following guidelines for performing neuromuscular exercises:

- **Frequency:** At least two days per week
- **Time:** At least 20 minutes per day
- **Intensity:** An effective intensity of neuromuscular exercise has not been determined.

Communicating Effectively During Training

Instructors must practice good communication in order to be effective. Communication serves a number of different purposes in fitness training, including the following:

- To establish trust
- To gain knowledge of medical, exercise and dietary history
- To establish the reasons for routines
- To motivate and encourage participants
- To explain how to perform certain movements

During training, instructors' communication must convey content (information, strategies), motivation and emotion. Receiving information (listening to clients and interpreting their feedback) is just as important as transmitting information. Real communication begins with welcoming the feelings and opinions of each person in the conversation. Communication is not just about talking and listening. Almost 70 percent of human communication is nonverbal. Instructors should work to develop the following communicative skills:

- Demonstrating knowledge that develops their credibility
- Listening
- Using clear language

- Using a positive approach
- Alternating instructional methods: Demonstrating movements as well as explaining them

During training, fitness instructors must select the form of communication most appropriate for members of the class, particularly if beginners are present.

Observing Physiological Changes

Regular exercise practice creates physiological changes in the body. Morphological and functional modifications occur as a result of adaptation to training stimuli. Instructors must take this progressive adaptation into account when setting exercises for different skill levels. Table 5.3 summarises the physiological changes induced by resistance and aerobic training. However, instructors should remember that the magnitude of these changes depends on how they manage and apply training variables.

Table 5.3   Main Physiological Changes Induced by Training

	Physiological change
Aerobic training (cardiovascular component)	(+) Heart size (+) Systolic volume (–) Resting and submaximal heart rate (+) Maximum cardiac output (+) Capillary density of heart and skeletal muscle (+) Mitochondrial density of skeletal muscle (+) Blood volume
Resistance training (neuromuscular component)	Transformation of IIx to IIa fibres Change in pennation angle (+) Size of muscle fibres (+) Cross-sectional area of muscle (+) Number of muscular fibres (+) Voluntary activation of fibres (recruitment) (+) Rate of neural impulses (+)Synchronisation of motor units (+) Agonist–antagonist coordination (–) Inhibitory reflexes (–) Mitochondrial density of skeletal muscle (+) Capillary density of heart and skeletal muscle

(+) = increase in; (–) = decrease in.
Baechle and Earle 2008; Fleck and Kraemer 2004; Philip 2009; Wilmore, Costill and Kenney 2008.

Applying the Principles of Training

Fitness improvements are based on the body's capacity to adapt to stress stimuli. Several rules govern this adaptation that must be considered for training design. These rules are usually called *principles of training* (Earle and Baechle 2004; Howley and Thompson 2012; Issurin 2010; Swain and Leutholtz 2007). This section reviews the main principles and presents some examples of how to apply them.

Overload

To achieve adaptation, the training stimulus goes beyond the level at which the body is normally stressed. That is, to produce an adaptation, participants must reach a new threshold of exercise tolerance. Table 5.4 shows some ways to use these components in cardiore-

Table 5.4   Applying Overload to Cardiorespiratory, Resistance and Flexibility Training Programmes

Component of training	Cardiorespiratory training	Resistance training	Flexibility training
Volume	• Time • Distance • Kilocalories • METs × min • Steps	• Repetitions • Sets • Work (load times repetitions) • Time (isometric training)	• Sets • Time • Repetitions
Intensity	• Velocity • Watts • % $\dot{V}O_2$max • % $\dot{V}O_2$reserve • % Maximum heart rate • % Heart rate reserve	• Load (kg) • % 1RM • Power • Maximum number of repetitions • % of maximum number of repetitions • Velocity	• Range of movement
Type of exercise/ method	• Continuous • Discontinuous (accumulated exercise) • Walking • Running • Swimming • Cycling • Stepping • Elliptical	• Closed/open chain • Unilateral/bilateral • Stable/instable • Free weight • Machines • Elastic band • Body weight	• Ballistic methods or bouncing • Dynamic or slow stretching • Static stretching • Proprioceptive neuromuscular facilitation (PNF)
Frequency	• Days per week		

spiratory, resistance and flexibility training. In exercise, overload is regulated with different training components or variables: intensity, volume, type or method of exercise and frequency.

Specificity

The type of change produced by exercise depends on the character-istics of the stress produced by training. That is, the characteristics of a type of exercise determine, for example, whether the adaptation is mainly cardiorespiratory or muscular. Some examples of this prin-ciple include the following:

- Resistance or flexibility training adaptations are specific to the muscular group activated by the movement being practiced.
- Cardiorespiratory performance is higher when the exercises in the tests are similar to those employed in the fitness training.
- Resistance training has minimal effects on cardiorespiratory performance and vice versa.

Progression

Progression refers to the need to continually and progressively increase demand on the body over time in order to improve fitness. Here are some examples of this principle:

- **Aerobic training.** The ACSM suggests gradually progressing exercise volume by adjusting exercise duration, frequency or intensity (Garber et al. 2011). In this regard, progression from accumulated loads of at least 10 minutes to longer bouts is also recommended (Murphy, Blair, and Murtagh 2009).
- **Resistance training.** Increasing repetitions per set, number of sets or load (2 to 10 percent) is recommended in order to maintain adaptive responses (Kraemer et al. 2002; Hass, Fei-genbaum, and Franklin 2001; Peterson et al. 2005).
- **Flexibility training.** The ACSM suggests increasing duration of stretches (Garber et al. 2011).
- **Neuromotor training.** Progressive inclusion of instability resis-tance training is a way to change resistance and balance stim-ulus, although it does compromise mechanical performance of muscular training (Anderson and Behm 2005). Instructors can increase difficulty in terms of balance by using perturbation training (Fitzgerald et al. 2002).

Regularity or Continuity

This principle is related to the component of training frequency. When physical conditioning is stopped or reduced, training-induced cardiorespiratory, metabolic, musculoskeletal and neuromotor adaptations are reversed to varying degrees over time (Garber et al. 2011). If too much time goes by between exercise sessions, the adaptation will be lost, and detraining will occur. In order to avoid detraining, sessions must be performed several times per week. Frequency recommendations are as follows:

- **Aerobic training:** 3 to 5 days per week (Garber et al. 2011)
- **Resistance training:** 2 or 3 days per week (Hass et al. 2001; Kraemer et al. 2002; Peterson et al. 2005)
- **Flexibility sessions:** at least 2 days per week (Garber et al. 2011)
- **Neuromotor training:** at least 2 days per week (Garber et al. 2011)

Individual Responsiveness

Although general adaptation tendencies exist for several exercise regimens, the magnitude of the effect of a particular training regimen can vary significantly among individuals, and some exercisers may not respond as expected (Garber et al. 2011).

Instructors should consider this principle by prescribing exercise intensity to suit individual participants. As presented in table 5.4, some commonly used methods include the following:

- **Aerobic training**
  - % $\dot{V}O_2$max
  - % $\dot{V}O_2$reserve
  - % maximum heart rate (HRmax)
  - % heart rate reserve (HRR)
- **Resistance training**
  - % 1RM
  - Maximum number of repetitions
  - % of maximum number of repetitions
  - % of maximum velocity
- **Flexibility**
  - Individual amplitude of movement
  - Individual range of movement (Issurin 2010)

Conclusion

A key point for achieving goals is to adjust the dose of exercise to meet individual characteristics. Instructors should know the effect of planned training on different physical capabilities for providing security and confidence in the process.

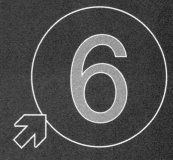

Preparing Fitness Programmes

Sonia García Merino
Susana Moral González

This chapter describes the basic requirements to consider before starting an exercise programme. To avoid unnecessary risks and offer their clients safe and effective exercise programmes, fitness instructors should clearly define programme objectives.

This chapter explores the following:

- Basic information to be gathered before starting any exercise programme
- Objectives and benefits of an exercise programme
- Level of fitness required to enroll in an exercise programme
- Restrictions on exercise (i.e., which people cannot participate)
- Different options for levels of intensity and impact

Gathering Information Prior to the Start of Class

Before starting an exercise programme, instructors should take into account a number of issues concerning safety and effectiveness. Gathering information on clients' health status, needs and objectives is of vital importance. Preparing a suitable environment or climate, establishing rapport and a high degree of credibility, providing client support and discovering clients' level of commitment (Griffin 1998) will enable instructors to grow closer to their clients. The initial interview allows clients to share information about their motivations, needs and desires.

Once instructors have established a positive relationship with their clients, they should collect information regarding the clients' medical history and relationship to exercise, which will allow them to do the following (ACSM 2009):

- Identify individuals with medical contraindications for exclusion from exercise programmes until those conditions have improved
- Recognise people with clinically significant diseases or conditions who should participate in a medically supervised exercise programme
- Detect individuals at increased risk for disease because of age, symptoms or risk factors who should undergo a medical evaluation and exercise testing before initiating an exercise programme or increasing the frequency, intensity or duration of their current programme
- Recognise special needs that may affect exercise testing and programming

For this purpose, clients should complete these forms or provide the following information (Heyward 2010):

- The PAR-Q (Physical Activity Readiness Questionnaire), designed by the Canadian Society for Exercise Physiology
- A medical history questionnaire with questions about personal health history
- Risk stratification of coronary heart disease
- Assessment of lifestyle
- Informed consent

The PAR-Q is a tool that detects which people may be at risk when starting an exercise programme. The validity of the PAR-Q questionnaire is specified for people between 15 and 69 years of age; people over 69 who are not physically active should be evaluated directly by a physician. It consists of seven questions. Clients who respond positively to any of the questions should be referred to a physician, who will verify that they may participate in the activity. These clients should also fill out the PARmed-X, which must be done by a physician. Pregnant women should complete a specific PARmed-X for Pregnancy form (Canadian Society for Exercise Physiology 2013).

Once the PAR-Q has been completed, instructors should ask clients for information regarding their personal health history, including medical diagnoses, past physical examinations, recent illness, orthopaedic problems, medication use, family history, exercise habits and caffeine, alcohol and tobacco use.

Instructors can use this information to analyse the client's level of risk, taking into account the following factors: age, family history, cigarette smoking, sedentary lifestyle, obesity, hypertension, dyslipidaemia and prediabetes. Next, instructors will set the risk level (low, moderate or high) and determine whether clients should receive a medical examination and clearance or an exercise test before beginning a physical activity or exercise programme. Clients may also need the supervision of a physician when participating in a maximal or submaximal exercise test (ACSM 2009).

The lifestyle assessment, on the other hand, provides valuable information that will help clients adhere to a fitness programme. Factors for success include family responsibilities, diet, occupation, type of residence and family support.

Before undergoing a physical fitness test or beginning a physical activity programme, clients must sign an informed consent form. This document outlines the risks and expected benefits of the programme or test.

Finally, after verifying the client's ability to participate in an exercise programme, in setting the corresponding objectives, instructors should consider three aspects: their client's wishes, the client's needs, and the probability that the activity will be integrated into the client's lifestyle. This allows instructors to propose realistic targets. For this, they should apply the five criteria of the SMART formula: A goal should be specific, measurable, accomplishment oriented, realistic and timed. This formula first appeared in a publication linked to the business world (Doran 1981), and it has been subsequently applied in different fields. These criteria will help participants achieve their goals more effectively.

Once instructors have determined that participants will be able to perform a programme safely and enthusiastically, they should take into account a number of practicalities prior to the workout. Before the session, instructors should monitor any new participants joining mid-programme or exercising for the first time. Another important aspect is knowledge of participants' previous experiences (gathered in the exercise history), which can influence exercise adherence; a person with a greater level of experience will have more realistic expectations than a beginner. In short, in order to have a successful and safe programme, instructors must have all the information concerning participants' health (e.g., previous injuries, fitness level and experience with exercise) before allowing them to begin the workout (use table 6.1 as a reference).

Programme Exercise Goals and Benefits

The objective of an exercise programme in this context is to improve the mental and physical health of the participants. Healthy people who want to maintain an optimal state of health will initially aim to improve health-related components of physical fitness, commonly defined as body composition, cardiorespiratory fitness, flexibility, muscular endurance and strength (USDHHS 1996) (see table 6.2).

Table 6.1   Five Criteria That Determine Client Objectives

Criteria	Objective
Specific	Objectives should be clear and specific enough to drive action. Effective use of questioning, probing and paraphrasing can help clients demonstrate the level of specificity they need in order to act.
Measurable	For many clients, being able to measure progress is an important incentive.
Accomplishment oriented	Stating objectives as accomplishments helps clients avoid leaping into action without knowing where they are going.
Realistic	An objective is realistic if the resources necessary to accomplish it are available, if it is under the client's control, and if clients make it a high priority.
Timed	A timed objective provides a powerful motivation for following an exercise programme.

Adapted from Griffin 1998.

Table 6.2   Health-Related Components of Physical Fitness

Component	Component definition
Cardiorespiratory fitness	Ability of the circulatory and respiratory systems to supply oxygen during sustained physical activity
Flexibility	Range of motion available at a joint
Muscular endurance	Ability of the muscle to continue to perform without fatigue
Strength	Ability of the muscle to exert force
Body composition	Relative amounts of muscle, fat, bone and other vital parts of the body

Based on U.S. Department of Health and Human Services 1996.

On the other hand, in relation to the quantity and quality of exercise, the ACSM's 2011 position stand includes a new component of health-related fitness, neuromotor fitness. Also called functional fitness training, this type of training incorporates exercises for balance, motor skills, coordination, agility and proprioceptive gait. Activities such as t'ai chi, yoga and qigong combine neuromotor, resistance and flexibility exercises.

Very strong scientific evidence shows that physically active people have higher levels of health-related fitness, a lower risk profile for developing a number of disabling medical conditions, and lower rates of various chronic diseases than people who are inactive (U.S. Department of Health and Human Services 2008). Participation in an exercise programme is clearly associated with health benefits, as summarised in table 6.3.

However, not only healthy people receive benefits from exercise programmes. Other populations, including pregnant or postpartum women, people with disabilities and overweight people, also benefit from exercise programmes.

The Physical Activity Guidelines Advisory Committee (2008) shows strong evidence indicating the following:

Table 6.3   Benefits of Engaging in an Exercise Programme

	Adults and older adults	Children and adolescents
Strong evidence	▪ Lowers risk of early death, coronary heart disease, stroke, high blood pressure, adverse blood lipid profile, type 2 diabetes, metabolic syndrome, colon cancer and breast cancer ▪ Prevents weight gains and falls, improves weight loss, cognitive function (for older adults) and cardiorespiratory and muscular fitness ▪ Reduces depression	▪ Improves cardiorespiratory and muscular fitness, bone health, cardiovascular and metabolic health biomarkers, and favourable body composition
Moderate to strong evidence	▪ Increases functional health (for older adults) and reduces abdominal obesity	
Moderate evidence	▪ Lowers risk of hip fracture, lung cancer and endometrial cancer ▪ Improves sleep quality and weight maintenance after weight loss ▪ Increases bone density	▪ Reduces symptoms of depression

Adapted from U.S. Department of Health and Human Services 2008.

■ Pregnant women in good health who perform moderate exercise increase their cardiorespiratory and metabolic fitness without putting the foetus at risk. In addition, participating in physical activity after giving birth does not appear to compromise breast milk volume or composition or the growth of the child.

■ Strong and moderate evidence exists that people with disabilities show significant improvements in cardiorespiratory fitness, strength and walking speed and distance. Limited data indicate improvements in flexibility, atherogenic lipids, bone mineral density and quality of life.

■ Overweight people receive the same health benefits from exercise as those who are not overweight. These benefits include lower rates of all-cause mortality, coronary heart disease, hypertension, stroke, type 2 diabetes, colon cancer and breast cancer. Adults of all sizes and shapes gain health and fitness benefits from habitual physical activity.

➡ ➡ ➡ Diseases and Conditions Requiring Permanent or Temporary Exercise Restrictions

Absolute contraindications
- Aortic aneurysm (dissecting)
- Aortic stenosis (severe)
- Congestive heart failure
- Crescendo angina
- Myocardial infarction (acute)
- Myocarditis (active or recent)
- Pulmonary or systemic embolism—acute
- Thrombophlebitis
- Ventricular tachycardia and other dangerous dysrhythmias (e.g., multifocal ventricular activity)
- Acute infectious disease (regardless of aetiology)

Relative contraindications
- Aortic stenosis (moderate)
- Subaortic stenosis (severe)
- Marked cardiac enlargement
- Supraventricular dysrhythmias (uncontrolled or high rate)
- Ventricular ectopic activity (repetitive or frequent)
- Ventricular aneurysm
- Hypertension—untreated or uncontrolled severe (systemic or pulmonary)
- Hypertrophic cardiomyopathy
- Compensated congestive heart failure

Programme Suitability

Most people benefit from exercise programmes. More and more studies show the importance of remaining active despite having medical complications. People with arthritis, cancer, diabetes, disabilities, dyslipidaemia, human immunodeficiency virus (HIV), hypertension, metabolic syndrome, osteoporosis, pulmonary disease, renal disease and so on may include physical exercise as a treatment for improving their physical condition and quality of life. Hardman and Stensel (2003) report strong evidence of this, and Pedersen and Saltin (2006) present the guidelines for exercise prescriptions.

However, exercise may present more risks than benefits to some people. The following list shows diseases or conditions that require permanent or temporary restriction until the condition has been treated or stabilised, or has passed the acute phase. These diseases are called absolute contraindications. Participants with relative

- Subacute, chronic or recurrent infectious diseases (e.g., malaria, others)
- Uncontrolled metabolic disorders (diabetes mellitus, thyrotoxicosis, myxedema)
- Complicated pregnancy (e.g., toxemia, hemorrhage or incompetent cervix)

Special prescriptive conditions
- Aortic (or pulmonary) stenosis—mild angina pectoris and other manifestations of coronary insufficiency (e.g., postacute infarct)
- Cyanotic heart disease
- Shunts (intermittent or fixed)
- Conduction disturbances: complete atrioventricular block, left bundle-branch block or Wolff-Parkinson-White syndrome
- Dysrhythmias—controlled
- Fixed-rate pacemakers
- Intermittent claudication
- Hypertension: systolic 160–180, diastolic 105+
- Chronic infections
- HIV
- Renal, hepatic and other metabolic insufficiency
- Obesity
- Single kidney
- Advanced pregnancy (late 3rd trimester)

Adapted from Canadian Society for Exercise Physiology 2002.

contraindications may need direct or indirect medical supervision of the exercise programme. Those who require a special prescriptive condition may need an individualised programme with medical monitoring or initial supervision.

Required Level of Fitness and Intensity and Impact Options

Modern exercise programmes are tailored to different population groups as well as for different fitness levels. By varying the intensity, volume and type of exercise, instructors can implement exercise programmes for people with very different characteristics and conditions. A participant's level of fitness and amount of exercise received through outside physical activity will determine the frequency, intensity and time employed in the exercise programme.

Exercise intensity is strongly linked to its benefits. Recent studies have supported the greater benefits of vigorous versus moderate exercise (ACSM 2011). The study by Swain and Franklin (2006) shows that if the total energy expenditure of exercise is held constant, exercise performed at a vigorous intensity appears to convey greater cardioprotective benefits than exercise of a moderate intensity. On the other hand, in another study whose purpose was to determine whether various intensities of aerobic training differentially affect aerobic capacity, Gormley et al. (2008) conclude that when volume of exercise is controlled, higher intensities of exercise are more effective for improving $\dot{V}O_2$max than lower intensities of exercise in healthy young adults. Moreover, the range of intensity at which participants must work to obtain the benefits seems to be based on their fitness level. These data should be interpreted with caution because exercise intensity must always be adapted to the needs of each participant.

The ACSM (2011) provides some recommendations in terms of intensity and type of exercise for each of the components of health-related fitness. These recommendations are covered in chapter 5, but they have been summarized here:

- **Cardiorespiratory exercise.** Moderate to vigorous intensity is recommended for most adults, and light- to moderate-intensity exercise may be beneficial for unconditioned people. Regular, purposeful exercise that involves major muscle groups is recommended.

- **Resistance exercise.** Intensity recommendations are as follows: 60 to 70 percent of 1RM (moderate to hard intensity) for novice to intermediate clients; 80 percent of 1RM (hard to very hard intensity) for experienced strength-trained clients; 40 to 50 percent of 1RM (very light to light intensity) for older people beginning exercise; 40 to 50 percent of 1RM (very light to light intensity) may be beneficial for improving strength in sedentary persons beginning a resistance training programme; 50 percent of 1RM (light to moderate intensity) is recommended for improving muscular endurance; 20 to 50 percent of 1RM is recommended for improving power in older adults. Resistance exercises involving each major muscle group are recommended.

- **Flexibility exercise.** Participants should stretch to the point of feeling tightness or slight discomfort. A series of flexibility exercises for each of the major muscle–tendon units is recommended. Static flexibility (active or passive), dynamic flexibility, ballistic flexibility and PNF are all effective.

- **Neuromotor exercise training.** An effective intensity of neuromotor exercise has not been determined. Exercises involving motor skills (e.g., balance, agility, coordination and gait), proprioceptive exercise training and multifaceted activities (e.g., tai chi, yoga) are recommended for older people to improve and maintain physical function and reduce falls in those at risk for falling. The effectiveness of neuromuscular exercise training in younger and middle-aged persons has not been established, but benefits are likely.

Conclusion

Safety and effectiveness in exercise programs should be a priority for fitness instructors. Although the benefits of exercise greatly exceed the risks, we must make every effort to minimize them, using the protocols for it. On the other hand, the approach of achievable goals tailored to the capabilities of customers ensure successful and healthy fitness programs.

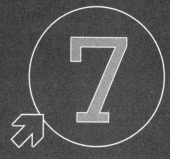

Delivering a Group Fitness Class

Simona Pajaujiene

Today, a variety of methods exist to help develop endurance, flexibility, strength and coordination of movements. However, exercises that don't engage the emotions get boring quickly, and exercising alone requires strong motivation. Therefore, joining a group of active like-minded people to perform diverse activities to music under the guidance of a professional fitness instructor can infuse an exercise routine with feeling and colour.

In addition to the physical, biochemical and physiological benefits of exercising, group fitness (GF) exercises provide mental and social benefits. They change the participants' relationship with themselves and their environment, encourage interaction, enhance communication skills and self-expression, and develop movement and sense of rhythm. Socialisation is a very important aspect of group fitness classes (GFCs). A lack of social support can be linked with an increased risk of many diseases and with early mortality (Barth et al. 2010; Kuper et al. 2006; Heather 2006; Clark 2005). Many forms of GFC can be organised in indoor or outdoor settings, and they can increase physical activity and social connectedness (McGonigal 2007). GFCs can offer opportunities for involvement to vulnerable, isolated or sensitive groups of people, such as seniors, pregnant women, mothers with babies and teenagers.

The aim of GFCs is to improve health-related fitness components and help people live healthier and happier lives through exercise (Kennedy and Yoke 2005). It is interesting to note that the current guidelines validate a typical group exercise class format dating back to the 1970s. These exercises develop the cardiovascular system's capacity, muscular strength and endurance and flexibility, and help participants maintain the most appropriate weight and body composition. Today, many group classes are also incorporating balance and agility exercises (Kennedy-Armbruster and Yoke 2009). The degree to which each component of fitness is developed can vary widely. For example, one person may have good cardiorespiratory endurance, but lack muscular strength. Another may be very strong, but lack flexibility. The overall goal of GFCs is to include all components of fitness in the programme, although they are not necessarily all included in one class (Kennedy and Yoke 2005). Body toning exercises put more emphasis on muscular strength and endurance and dance or cycling exercises work on cardiovascular system's capacity, whereas stretching exercises put more stress on flexibility.

Helping Clients Choose Group Fitness Classes

Offering a variety of class times and activities is important for successful fitness programmes. Of course, instructors should keep in mind that the effectiveness of GF exercises (as well as of any other physical activity) depends on the proper choice of exercise, as well as their frequency, intensity and duration. When choosing the type and intensity of exercises, it is necessary to evaluate a client or participant's fitness and exercising objectives. Exercising improperly or choosing loads that are too high may lead to negative effects and cause injuries, illnesses, fatigue or exhaustion.

GFCs can be adapted for different kinds of people. Some classes are more suitable for school children, students, people with lower physical fitness levels (beginners), people who are overweight or those with movement and health limitations. Classes conducted at a high intensity level are suited for sporty, active men and women. Regardless of their needs and preferences, participants can find a GFC that suits them. Such classes will be far more effective and useful. GFC choice often depends on the personalities and professionalism of fitness instructors and managers working at sport clubs. Large clubs should plan their schedules so that participants can choose exercise classes according to their needs and preferences. All GFCs can be divided into several subgroups (table 7.1):

- In accordance with a health-related fitness component (so that instructors can easily choose and develop necessary or weaker physical characteristics)
- In accordance with the difficulty of choreography (Since many group exercises do not require knowledge of dance basics, they may seem attractive to people who do not like dance or do not feel eurhythmics.)
- In accordance with the needs or hobby of a client

Table 7.1 Subgroups of Group Fitness Classes

Group fitness class objective	Examples of group fitness classes
According to health-related fitness components	
Muscular strength and endurance	Body toning, group stability ball, circuit strength training, functional training.
Cardiorespiratory endurance	Combo or low impact, step aerobics, dance (hip-hop, Latin, funk), indoor cycling, rowing, kickboxing
Flexibility (*mind and body*)	Stretching, Pilates, yoga, t'ai chi
Fusion classes (*muscular and cardiorespiratory endurance*)	Cardio core, interval training, step and pump, cycle strength, aqua fitness
According to choreography to music	
Non-choreographed classes	Body toning, functional training, circuit training, indoor cycling, rowing, yoga, Pilates, aqua fitness*, Fitball*, kickboxing*
Choreographed classes	High impact, low impact, step aerobics, dance (Latin, hip-hop)
According to need and hobby	
Lifestyle-based physical activity	Outdoor walking, Nordic walking, in-line skating, cycling, boot camp, sport conditioning
Dance-based class	Zumba, Nia, funk, Latin dance, country dancing
Equipment-based cardiorespiratory training	Treadmill, rowing, cross-country skiing, elliptical machines, slide training, Bosu balance
Martial art classes	Boxing, kickboxing, Kendo
Special groups	Classes for seniors, children, people with obesity, back problems and other medical limitations, pregnant women and mothers with babies

*Subject to the methodology applied by the fitness instructor; these exercises can be attributed to both choreographed and non-choreographed exercises.

GF exercises can be adapted to any skill level because they don't involve competition. Clients who want to participate in GFCs should move from low-intensity, low-impact sessions to more strenuous sessions using target heart rate (THR) as a guide. Further, they should take introductory classes (for step, kickboxing or other specialised forms of aerobics) to develop the skills needed for participation in the regular classes. Instructors should help participants choose the type of workout that is right for them. The physical fitness and health of each person is different; therefore, workouts should meet the expectations and needs of each client (table 7.2).

The most important recommendations are as follows:

- GFC frequency: Up to 60 minutes per day, two to five days per week
- Participants should choose more than one type of GFC (e.g., dance or yoga) so that they exercise all health-related fitness components (i.e., the cardiovascular system's capacity, muscular strength and endurance as well as flexibility) throughout the week. For example, they could do two workouts for strengthening the cardiovascular system (e.g., cycling exercises, climbing exercises) plus one or two workouts for strengthening and stretching muscles (e.g., body toning, Pilates, yoga).
- Participants should choose exercises according to their physical fitness level, rather than based on the advice of friends or their admiration of a certain instructor.
- The load should not be too great (numerous workouts in a row are not recommended, unless the load is partly combined with exercising in a gym). For example, after doing cycling exercises, participants may do a few series of exercises strengthening the upper body in a gym, or prior to doing a stretching or yoga exercise, they may do a 30-minute workout for aerobic load.

Table 7.2   General Recommendations When Choosing a Group Fitness Class

Characteristics of participants	Examples of group fitness classes
Beginners	Body toning, functional training, walking, cycling, Pilates, aqua fitness and other classes, if they are indicated as suitable for the beginners
Overweight people	Aqua fitness, group stability ball, Pilates, yoga, low impact, body toning, circle training, cycling, walking, functional training
People suffering from obesity and joint problems	Aqua fitness, group stability ball, Pilates, yoga, functional training

Core Concepts in Class Design

For the most favourable conditions, each GF workout, regardless of its type, should maintain the recommended structure. This allows instructors to include all health-related fitness components in a single workout. A GFC should consist of four parts:

- Warm-up (7 to 15 minutes)
- Cardiorespiratory activity (20 to 30 minutes)
- Muscular conditioning (10 to 20 minutes)
- Flexibility exercises and cool-down (7 to 10 minutes)

These segments are aligned with the health-related fitness components provided by the American College of Sports Medicine (ACSM 2009), and they apply to most types of GF classes. However, there is no strict standard or workout format because different exercises may vary in duration, order, choice of exercises and their constitutive parts. Different movements and equipment can be used to warm up depending on the class (techniques for step, Fitball, indoor cycling, aqua and Pilates all differ). Cardiorespiratory activity is not performed in stretching or in yoga classes and muscular conditioning is not performed in dance classes. The nature of the cool-down and flexibility portion also depends on the class. Body toning classes require longer sessions of more serious stretching. In water classes, the cool-down and stretching portion should be short because of the water temperature and body thermoregulation. GF instructors can determine their own rules for the duration, intensity and choice of exercises in their classes.

Warm-Up

A warm-up should do the following:

- Psychologically prepare for the workout (motivate the participants and help them focus their attention)
- Physiologically prepare for the workout (increase cardiac activity and prepare body systems for a more intensive workout)
- Prevent injuries

For gradual progression, the programme should begin with low-impact movements and dynamic stretching for the whole body (Howley and Franks 2007). Participants do various well-known, simple exercises for the hands, shoulders, waist and legs. Warm-up exercises should be repeated more than once. Movements are small at the beginning, but range of movement increases as the body warms up. Instructors often use this time to introduce *rehearsal moves*, or movements that will be included during the aerobic part of the workout (Appel 2007). Instructors should lead participants through exercises at a moderate pace, gradually increasing load intensity (up to 60 percent of maximum cardiac system activity) to increase muscle and core temperatures without causing fatigue (Baechle and Earle 2008).

The following factors determine duration and choice of exercises as well as intensity of the warm-up:

- Fitness level and age of the group (advanced or beginners; adults or young people)
- Ambient temperature (cold or hot)
- Time of the day (morning or evening)

Beginners, participants in morning classes and those working out in a cool environment will benefit from a longer, more intentional warm-up. The following errors may contribute to a poor warm-up:

- The instructor does not make contact with the group.
- Participants try to warm up as quickly as possible instead of gradually increasing load intensity.
- Movements are too intense (hops) or complex (with twists).
- Movements involve changes of direction or long combinations.
- Instructor does not provide rehearsal moves.
- The warm-up is too intense, leading to group fatigue.
- Stretching is improperly carried out or is incomplete.
- Music is too fast.

Cardiorespiratory Activity

The aim of this portion of the workout is to develop the cardiovascular system's capacity as well as other physical properties. This part takes up to 30 minutes, which is the period of time for the amount of aerobic activity required to have a positive effect on the cardiovascular system. Depending on the specificity of training, the duration of the aerobic portion may vary (15 to 40 minutes).

This part is specific to the type of class. Movements should concentrate on the large muscles of the body, and instructors should incorporate repetitive and rhythmic motions (and combinations of the two) into the routines. Basic steps and upper body moves elevate the heart rate to within the target zone. Instructors can individualise the style (e.g., calisthenics workout, Latin dance, or running or cycling routine).

Possible errors that may contribute to a poor cardiorespiratory activity segment include the following:

- Intensity is too high or too low.
- The workout content does not correspond to the workout type.
- Choreography is too complex or too dull, or includes too many repetitive moves.
- The instructor does not offer alternatives for moves that are either very complex or simple.
- Muscle load is uneven (i.e., one foot dominates in the steps).
- Pulse is not counted.
- Instructor does not have strong communication and leadership skills.
- Music is inappropriate for the routine's movements or the participants' skill level.

A 3- to 5-minute active, standing transition should follow the cardiorespiratory segment. The aim is to gradually decrease the load and restore normal breathing rate and functioning of circulatory system. During this part, instructors lead participants through smaller and slower movements that prepare the body for muscular strength and endurance building exercises. Instructors encourage participants to relax, slow down, keep their arms at or below heart level and use less effort to perform movements. Instructors should play slower music and use a calm tone of voice as they lead the class through calm, rhythmic movements or simple walking exercises with attention to the breath (Kennedy-Armbruster and Yoke 2009).

Muscular Conditioning

The aim of this type of exercise is to increase endurance, to strengthen joints, ligaments and major muscle groups or simply to enhance the body's composition and appearance. Participants can use additional resistance devices (e.g., weights, bands or steps) and can perform exercises while standing, kneeling or lying down. These activities usually begin in the standing position and gradually move to the floor for abdominal and back strengthening exercises, which many instructors use to end their classes. The duration and content of this part highly depends on the type of exercise in the main aerobic part. It can be completely omitted if, for example, the workout has already covered body toning or strength training exercises.

Possible errors that contribute to a poor muscular conditioning segment include the following:

- Participants have improper posture and use incorrect movement technique.
- The choice of exercises does not correspond to the participants' fitness level (i.e., the instructor does not present modifications to make movements simpler or more complex).
- Exercises load muscle groups that were worked heavily during the main part of the workout.
- Instructors spend this time strengthening their own muscles rather than noticing the group's work and errors.
- Music is so loud that it keeps participants from concentrating on the exercises.

Flexibility Exercises and Cool-Down

The aim of this portion is to do the following:

- Further lower the heart rate
- Clear muscles from accumulated by-products of the oxidation process (lactate, urea)
- Help muscle fibres return to their original functional and biochemical condition
- Avoid muscular imbalances and incorrect body posture due to muscle shortening after session
- Increase muscle flexibility and joint mobility
- Decrease the risk of injuries
- Help participants relax and calm down

The final cool-down provides an opportunity for body systems to gradually return to preexercise levels. GFCs consist mainly of static stretches, which are usually performed either lying or sitting on the floor. The stretches are held for at least 10 seconds. The harder and more intense the workout, the longer the stretching procedure of individual muscle groups must be. Instructors should incorporate stretches for every muscle group, especially those specifically worked on during the class, and should focus on the hamstrings and lower back. Stretching can be combined with relaxation and breathing exercises.

Possible errors that contribute to a poor flexibility and cool-down session include the following:

- Stretching exercises are performed too quickly, failing to retain the position or concentrate on the muscle being stretched.
- Stretching is too intense and painful.

- Participants hold their breath while stretching.
- Instructors lead class in high-risk exercises or competitive strategy (Who can reach the farthest?).
- The cool-down decreases impact and intensity too quickly
- Participants or instructors show off their gymnastic skills.

Overall Guidelines

Instructors must follow these principles when conducting group fitness workouts:

- Always start workouts with a warm-up and gradually increase the intensity of movements.
- Choose exercises for the aerobic part of the session that will allow participants to work at an optimal physical load.
- Finish the aerobic part of the workout with a cool-down.
- Lead participants through strengthening exercises for the major muscle groups (particularly those in the abdomen and back).
- Finish the workout with stretching and relaxation exercises.

Modifications to Planned Exercises

A professional and competent GF instructor must have knowledge of the following:

- Basics of anatomy, biomechanics and safety
- Peculiarities and possibilities of using additional inventory
- A great variety of exercises for individual muscle groups (from the most simple to the most complex)

During GFCs, instructors should lead the workout and observe the load intensity and performance of the whole group. If instructors notice group members showing signs of fatigue or performing exercises incorrectly, they should make the exercise easier or replace it, or simply advice those participants to rest. Instructors must observe all the participants as they exercise and then suggest modifications or other exercises according to the fitness level of each student.

Instructors should focus on participants and quickly respond to complaints or problems that arise during the workout. For example, if participants complain that their wrists hurt, the instructor should recommend a modification (e.g., perform the exercise on their fists to keep the wrist straight). If that does not help, the instructor can switch to another exercise. Instructors should choose exercises that are appropriate for the majority of participants, but also prepare simpler and more complex alternatives.

In general, GF instructors should observe and assist their participants and move around the group so that all students can see demonstrations. They should show empathy for participants, modifying any problematic exercises.

Incorporating Functional Exercise Progression

Progression refers to the process of progressively loading the body's systems and increasing the training stimulus over time to increase fitness adaptations gradually. Depending on the type of training, changing the variables of frequency, intensity, duration and mode can gradually make muscles stronger, build endurance and enhance neuromuscular control, coordination and balance (Kennedy 2003). This issue is very important to group exercise because instructors have to decide what exercises they are going to teach in their classes. The progressive functional training continuum (FTC) (Kennedy 2003; Yoke and Kennedy 2004) helps instructors make better decisions for their participants (figure 7.1) by suggesting exercises from easiest to hardest. The FTC ranks the exercises for a particular muscle group according to their difficulty level. Participants who have trouble performing an exercise can do an easier and safer modification. By gradually improving their strength and endurance, they will be able to perform harder exercises.

Less-skilled exercises are relatively easy to explain, and they don't involve balance or (as the name implies) require much skill. Such exercises are low risk and generally safe for almost all populations. Many of these exercises require isolation movements instead of total body movements and strengthen individual muscle groups.

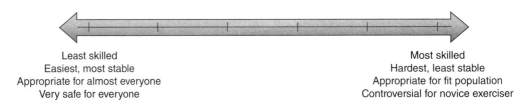

Least skilled	Most skilled
Easiest, most stable	Hardest, least stable
Appropriate for almost everyone	Appropriate for fit population
Very safe for everyone	Controversial for novice exerciser

Figure 7.1 Progressive functional training continuum.

Reprinted, by permission, from C. Kennedy-Armbruster and M. Yoke, 2014, *Methods of group exercise instruction,* 3rd ed. (Champaign, IL: Human Kinetics), 48.

Highly skilled exercises are harder to perform and less stable, and they require more skill in order to maintain joint integrity and core stability. Although these challenging exercises pose a greater risk, a very fit person with excellent core stability should be able to perform them safely and appropriately. Kennedy and Yoke (2005) suggested that GF instructors use the following model to choose which exercises will be safe for the whole class (table 7.3). Exercises 1 through 4 are most appropriate for group classes. Exercises 5 and 6 are better reserved for advanced classes or personal training.

GF instructors must weigh the risk of performing the exercise in its original form against the benefits. If the risk outweighs the benefits, they should select another exercise.

Intensity and Impact Options in Group Fitness Exercise

High loads often have a negative effect on the human body; taxing the heart, joints and tendons can lead to damage. However, choosing an appropriate physical load for group classes may help participants to achieve their goal of improved health. During the cardio part of GFCs, instructors can control the level of exertion in various ways (reducing or increasing the level of loading intension). They can increase

Table 7.3 Principles of the Progressive Functional Training Continuum

Steps	Description
1. Isolate and educate	Focus on isolating muscles and contracting individual muscles.
2. Add external resistance	Use external weights, elastic bands or tubes, increasing lever length.
3. Add functional training positions	Progress to a more functional body position (to sitting or standing).
4. Combine increased function and resistance	Overload the core stabiliser muscle in functional positions and maximise resistance from gravity, weights or bands.
5. Use multiple muscle groups with increased resistance and core challenge	Use multiple muscle groups and joint actions simultaneously or in combination; progress resistance, balance, coordination and torso stability.
6. Add balance, speed and rotational movements	Increase functional challenge by balancing on one leg, using a stability ball or applying plyometric movements, spinal rotation or some other sport-specific manoeuvre or life skill.

intensity by choosing more difficult steps or movements, raising and lowering the body's centre of gravity, adding high-impact movements, adding larger radial movements of arms and legs or increasing the pace. On the other hand, they can reduce the intensity by simplifying all of these elements. See the following list for suggestions on varying workout intensity.

Methods for Adjusting (Increasing or Decreasing) Workout Intensity

- Alter leverage length of limbs
- Alter amplitude of moves
- Alter the speed of moves (rhythm, rhythm variations)
- Alter the impact of moves (high or low)
- Alter the level of effort (level of exertion, muscle contraction)
- Alter the number of repetitions of moves
- Apply indoor equipment (e.g., bands, dumbbells, weighted bars or balls)
- Apply outdoor equipment (e.g., stairs, benches or hills)
- Change the place of workout (walking longer distances)

In addition to putting stress on the cardiovascular system (CVS), exercise also strains the musculoskeletal system. Increasing strain on the CVS also increases the strain on the skeleton and the muscles' need for oxygen.

Instructors need to know a variety of steps and moves as well as how to modify them into high- and low-impact steps according to the situation. The word *impact* in this instance means 'bouncing stress'. Low-impact exercises generally reduce stress on the joints (and spinal column) and high-impact ones increase the level of stress. For example, a grapevine step can be performed as a low-impact (as usual), high-impact (jump from one foot to the other) or combination (jump on the final fourth beat) exercise. During low-impact versions at least one foot remains on the ground, but during high-impact versions both feet leave the ground briefly (a small flight phase). The phrases *low impact* and *high impact* do not always reflect the intensity of training. Low-impact steps with large ranges of movements and long leverage can be more intense than high-impact movements, which are small and supple (Howley and Franks 2007).

It is important to understand that the physiological impact is not necessarily the same as the psychological or complexity impact. A workout that consists of simple combinations of moves and easy techniques can be quite intense in terms of the functioning of the cardiac system or oxygen or calorie consumption. Ironically, an extremely technical and complex workout with lots of intricate steps, exercises and hand moves may reduce the intensity, because participants have to pay close attention to the movements and try not to make mistakes.

Responding to a Medical Emergency

Everybody knows that exercising is beneficial and healthful; however, only few consider the idea that exercising may be harmful or unsafe. GF instructors must be prepared to safely handle an emergency medical situation. Inappropriate exercises, incorrect technique, disproportionate load and other external factors may lead to undesirable results. The following factors increase risk of injury:

- Too much activity
- Movements that are too fast
- Quick changes in directions
- Increased focus on the same muscle groups
- Lack of proper adaptation to the environmental conditions (extreme heat or cold)
- Lack of (or imbalance in) muscle strength
- Poor joint flexibility
- Poor cardiorespiratory fitness
- Obesity and specific medical problems (e.g., asthma or diabetes)

GF instructors should be aware of these risks and seek to control factors that increase the chances of injury. Advanced planning, training in injury recognition and emergency care, adequate equipment and facilities and counselling in activity selection all help reduce the possibility of injury.

Each health club should familiarise clients with the safety rules of exercise in order to avoid unpleasant surprises (e.g., chronic traumas, injuries or illnesses). Therefore instructors should give the following recommendations to participants in their fitness classes:

- Prior to exercising (and periodically), participants should check their health.
- Participants should not exercise while experiencing illness symptoms or residual effects of trauma.
- Instructors should recommend control in regard to exercise technique (i.e., do not try to do as much as possible; rather try to do the exercise as correctly as possible).

- Participants should follow the methodology of exercising (some clients cut out stretching to shorten workout time).

- Instructors should choose appropriate load intensity or additional load (e.g., step height or weight lifted).

- Instructors should choose a universal (or recommended) exercising schedule and try to follow it.

- Participants should wear appropriate workout clothing and footwear (e.g., for exercising outdoors, wear clothing that offers protection from the sun, cold or wind).

- Participants should drink sufficient amounts of liquid during and after the workout and eat nutritious food.

Educating participants about the proper intensity of the exercise session (how to stay in the THR zone) and how to recognise the signs and symptoms of overuse helps reduce risk of injury. GF instructors must be very attentive to their groups and respond to various warning signs (e.g., change of face colour, breathing, movement or tone of voice). They must inform their clients about the bodily signs and sensations that indicate serious illnesses.

Participants must stop exercising and seek medical attention if they experience any of the following warning signs:

- Unusual fatigue
- Nausea
- Dizziness
- Chest tightness or any pain in the area from the jaw to the waist
- Uncontrollable muscles
- Severe suffocation
- Allergic reactions (e.g., rash)
- Visual impairment

Accidents and Sudden Illnesses

The fitness environment has the potential to be dangerous. Fitness centres must develop emergency action plans that guide their procedures in the event of accident or incident (Howley and Franks 2007). These plans are specific to the environment (e.g., pool, group fitness hall, outdoor area). Examples of medical emergencies include heart attacks, strokes and injuries incurred through poor technique, mistakes with equipment or lack of concentration. All employees must receive staff training.

The effects of a sudden illness or an accident may cause the body's structure and function to change. The general role of GF instructors in an emergency can be described with the acronym CALM:

Calm yourself

Assess the situation

Locate assistance if available

Make the area safe

Staff members should call emergency services in the following situations:

- Casualty is unconscious
- They feel unable to handle the situation themselves
- The casualty's condition is worsening
- They suspect any of the following:
  - Fractures or severe dislocations
  - Head, neck or spine injury
  - Severe external bleeding
  - Internal injuries
  - Serious medical problems (heart attack, asthma or diabetic emergencies)

Responsibilities of a Group Fitness Instructor

Instructors have a distinct relationship with the group and each individual participant; their interpersonal skills and other professional competencies must be evident.

- Excellent instructors radiate positive energy, which helps participants feel livelier, stronger and more open and energetic.
- Excellent instructors work with joy and inspiration, and focus on people, rather than on their images in a mirror.
- Their own image, mood, thoughts and actions are the instructors' responsibility. Their posture, face and speech highly influence clients. Knowing this, instructors must organise their personal lives accordingly: eating healthy food, getting adequate rest, preparing for workouts in advance, regenerating spiritually and conveying optimism.
- Instructors are leaders, but they should not place themselves on an unattainable pedestal. They should not be afraid to make mistakes. Participants like to know that their instructor is also an ordinary person; this will lead them to become more open and ask more questions.
- Moreover, instructors should do the following:
  - Be punctual (should not run into the room at the last minute)

- Look professional (set an example to clients through their clothing)
- Have excellent communication skills (should be assertive, yet encouraging and affirming, making participants feel important and accepted for who they are)

Instructors will achieve professional excellence by dedicating themselves to their work and nurturing their spirit:

- Instructors should have knowledge of anatomy, physiology and kinesiology and should be able to provide first aid, if necessary. They need to fully understand the effects of each exercise on the body and determine the intensity of chosen exercises.
- Instructors must regularly participate in seminars and courses (both dedicated to their speciality, and those for healthy lifestyle, psychology and pedagogy), read relevant literature, watch videos and co-operate with colleagues.

High professional requirements are set for GF instructors. Due to the specificity of exercising (i.e., continuous conducting techniques) they must be able to do the following:

- Choose the correct exercises and give instructions for step combinations (according to the principle 'from simple to more complex, from known to unknown')
- Perform exercises technically and flawlessly, logically and consistently move from one exercise to another, make connections among exercises and rhythmically coordinate them with the music, if necessary, all while maintaining a positive mood
- Comment on the exercises, noting their purpose and drawing attention to important technical details
- Modify exercises or combinations of steps that are too complex (e.g., respond to needs of participants, adapt movements to the fitness level of clients, provide alternatives)
- Demonstrate exercises from various positions (facing participants and presenting a mirror image, standing with their back to participants and offering a side view) to help participants understand movements
- Observe the participants during exercise and correct any mistakes (indicate mistakes generally so that the people making the error do not feel uncomfortable; if they fail to respond to the prompt, approach them or explain the errors after the workout)
- Follow workout intensity and pulse changes, and adjust physical load as needed

- Encourage a positive mood among participants
- Use various verbal or audible signals to prompt participants
- Change location during the workout (i.e., do not stand in front of the group all the time, but move to the centre or side) and approach beginners or participants who want help
- Maintain ability to perform various exercises and moves (i.e., be in good physical condition), and cultivate an excellent musical ear

Requirements Set for Instructors:

- Prepare the room (depending on the club's job descriptions, this may include ventilation, cleanliness and order)
- Prepare for workouts ('What will I do and how?' Plan the essential scheme of a class and choose music)
- Wear clean and tidy clothing
- Comply with hygiene requirements (e.g., have clean hair and nails and fresh breath) and look appropriate for a fitness setting (long coloured nails, loose hair, excessive jewellery and bright makeup are not appropriate during a workout)
- Use a simple speech style; offer clear and brief instructions and comments
- Listen to participants' needs, but gradually make them do what is necessary and useful
- Pay particular attention to beginners
- Send anyone who is ill home or to a doctor
- Avoid discussing diseases, illnesses, politics, religion and crime with clients
- Avoid making up answers to a question (instead, instructors should promise to look into it)
- Create a sense of connection among group members (e.g., organise tea parties, create traditions and rituals)
- Start with the easier exercises and steps, then combine them and increase length and difficulty (i.e., shift from simple to more complex movements, from known to unknown)
- Use various verbal and audible signals
- Try to make participants feel welcome and well liked
- Take responsibility for their work

Instructors should establish, publicise and maintain standards of ethical behaviour in fitness settings, and inform and protect members of the public and customers using the services of exercise professionals (www.ereps.eu.com). GF instructors should behave in a positive and constructive manner. Several organisations have outlined ethical practice guidelines and developed basic exercise standards for the field of group exercise (IDEA 2005; AFAA 2002).

Ethical Practice Guidelines for Group Fitness Instructors (IDEA 2005)

- Always be guided by the best interests of the group, while acknowledging individuals.
- Provide a safe exercise environment.
- Obtain the education and training necessary to lead group exercise.
- Use truth, fairness and integrity to guide all professional decisions and relationships.
- Maintain appropriate professional boundaries.
- Uphold a professional image through conduct and appearance.

The *Code of Ethical Practice* defines good practice for professionals in the fitness industry by reflecting on the core values of rights, relationships, responsibilities and standards. Instructors should also respect any specific laws and requirements of the country they work in. The European Register of Exercise Professionals (EREPS), regulated by the EuropeActive (formerly European Health and Fitness Association [EHFA] Standards Council, outlined the Code's four principles:

Rights: Exercise professionals will be respectful of their customers and of their rights as individuals.

Relationships: Exercise professionals will nurture healthy relationships with their customers and with other health professionals.

Personal responsibilities: Exercise professionals will demonstrate and promote a clean and responsible lifestyle.

Professional standards: Exercise professionals will seek to adopt the highest level of professional standards in their work and the development of their career (www.ereps.eu).

Conclusion

In this chapter, we have focused on the recommendation for choosing GFCs and core concepts in class design. We have listed main guidelines for successful leading and possible errors that contribute to a poor class delivering in each segment. We also covered safety issues incorporating functional exercise progression, intensity adjustment methods and emergency medical situation in GF workouts.

Group exercise has established itself as one of the attractive physical activities offered in fitness clubs, centers and studios. As you noticed, though, they are not the best or only valuable method or class type for fitness improvement. Many alternative forms of GFCs have been developed over the last 30 years. While some classes are more popular than others, we can't forget to integrate the health components of fitness into each GF class so that clients can enjoy the benefits. GF exercise programs must be individualized as much as possible by considering general principles in relation to information about participant health and physical fitness status. Ongoing recommendations and modifications for exercise should be made to ensure that participants' programs remain appropriate and safe.

Besides being positive role models, instructors also need to establish a comfortable environment for participants. GF instructors must know professional requirements and responsibilities and maintain standards of ethical behaviour in fitness settings. One of the biggest challenges for the group exercise instructor is balancing all of these elements. The information discussed in this chapter is fundamental for a skilled group exercise leader, and we highly recommend that all instructors develop their abilities in this important area.

Teaching Group Fitness to Music

Rita Santos Rocha

Nuno Pimenta

Music plays a very important role in motivating the participants and helping the instructor conduct the class. It is a tool for the instructor, if used properly. Besides setting an uplifting mood, music also plays several important technical roles in fitness classes, including controlling the speed of movements and ensuring continuity of exercise throughout the session.

Characteristics of Music
Used in Fitness Classes

The music used in fitness classes can be a determinant for the motivation levels in those classes, and therefore should be adjusted to the client's profile. For example, music from the 60's is usually more appreciated by clients that were born by then (Karageorghis and Priest, 2012, pp. 59). On the other hand, the selection of music could be based on cultural factors. Music selection is an important feature instructors should address properly because it helps instructors control various aspects of a class (e.g., speed of movement or number of repetitions of a specific exercise). For this purpose, music used in fitness classes must have specific characteristics to be suited for different types of clients and classes. Specific fitness activities sometimes demand specific music selections as well. Such characteristics include

- music speed,
- music continuum and
- music structure.

Music Speed

Music speed, as measured by the number of beats per minute (BPM), is a major issue when teaching group fitness classes to music. It determines the speed of movement and correlates with the class difficulty level. Increasing or decreasing the BPM raises or lowers the class difficulty level, respectively. Music's BPM influences class difficulty level in terms of two factors:

- **Complexity.** When the BPM is high, participants can perform more movements per minute, which increases the session's complexity.
- **Intensity.** Raising the speed at which movements are executed in a cardio workout (by raising music's BPM) increases both the metabolic intensity and difficulty level of the class.

Of course, many other aspects can influence either the complexity or intensity of a workout.

Music Continuum

Music continuum refers to music that it is uninterrupted, which is helpful as a reference for movement repetition at all times during group fitness classes. This means that the fitness instructor does not have to count the number of repetitions or set the tempo or movement speed. Therefore the fitness instructor is free to perform other tasks during the class, such as correcting participant performance, motivating the class or maintaining a positive atmosphere. In a recent review, Karageorghis et al. (2012, pp. 47) state that 'the use of music has been found to yield ergogenic effects in the exercise domain while also promoting psychological (e.g., enhanced affect) and psychophysical (reduced ratings of perceived exertion) benefits'.

In order to take full advantage of using music in group fitness classes, the instructor must learn the structure of the chosen music and specially prepare to use it in class.

Music Structure

Music for group fitness classes has a very specific structure that is extremely useful for helping fitness instructors facilitate their tasks because it is predictable. This structure includes the following aspects:

- Beat
- Metre
- Musical eight
- Musical phrase

Beat

The *beat* is the basic unit of time in music. It sets the music's speed (tempo), as figured in beats per minute (BPM). Music is divided into bars, organised by tempo and metre. Stronger and weaker beats help to set the music's style by determining the music's rhythm, which is different from the music's tempo. Rhythm in music is characterised by a repeating sequence of stronger (downbeats and on-beats) and weaker beats (upbeats). Downbeats are particularly important because most movements performed to music in a group fitness class start on the first beat (also called a *master downbeat*; see chapter 9). Downbeats fall on odd numbered counts and upbeats are even numbered, as seen in figure 8.1.

Metre

Most often, music follows a repeated pattern that allows us to identify a rhythm, which is called the *metre*. Common patterns include triple metre, used in waltz music, and quadruple metre, which is often used in electronic dance music. Music with quadruple metre is most often used for group fitness classes, and it has a repeating pattern containing four beats, where the first odd-numbered beat is the downbeat and the third beat is also strong, though not as strong as the downbeat, and is called the on-beat, while the even-numbered beats are upbeats (figure 8.2).

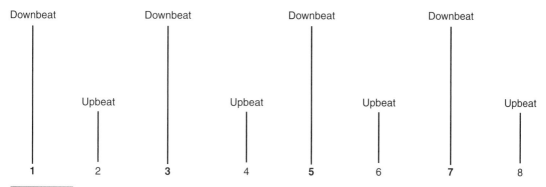

Figure 8.1 Downbeats and upbeats in an eight-beat sequence.

Musical Eight

The *musical eight* is a popular concept in choreographed activities, but is also a musical structure. In quadruple-metre music prepared for group fitness classes, it is possible to identify two sets of four beats that go together to form a sequence of eight consecutive beats: the musical eight. Here, the first beat, or master downbeat, is stronger than the following seven beats (figure 8.3).

Musical Phrase

A *musical phrase* is determined by both the music's melody and its beats. This means that a musical phrase is distinguished by the previous and the following phrases, by the instruments playing, by any lyrics sung and even by the rhythm. For music used in and specially prepared for group fitness classes, it is possible to identify a fixed pattern of musical phrases: Groups of four consecutive musical eights (4 × 8 beats) constitute a musical phrase. This means that

Downbeat

On-beat

Upbeat   Upbeat

1   2   3   4

Figure 8.2 Beats in a quadruple metre.

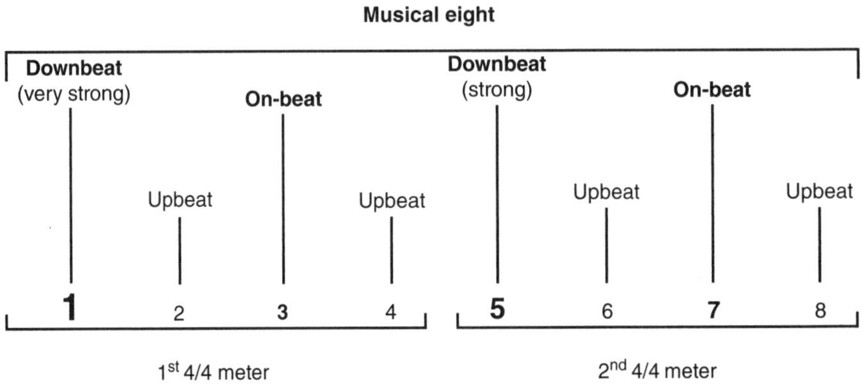

Musical eight

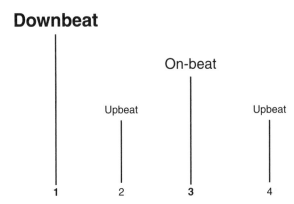

Figure 8.3 Beats in a musical eight.

in every 32 beats, it is possible to identify a new instrument, a new lyric, a different rhythm or simply the chorus. Because of this phrase pattern, instructors should prepare all classes and choreographies for a 32-beat musical phrase. Although some quadruple-metre music may use 16- or 64-beat phrases, they will not pose a problem for 32-beat choreography.

Moving to the Beat

As stated before, fitness music has a specific tempo, determined by BPM and adapted to each activity that sets the movement cadence (i.e., the velocity at which the movements are performed).

Different activities require adapted cadences of movement. For instance, when the Step Reebok programme was launched, a stepping rate of 118 to 128 BPM (118 BPM = 29.5 cycles per minute; 128 BPM = 32 cycles per minute) was recommended. A few years later, many step routines were being performed at faster cadences, such as 135 BPM or even faster. The current stepping rate is set by music that can be adjusted from 125 to 150 BPM; 125 BPM is considered a slow cadence that is proper for use with beginners, elderly people, pregnant women, and people with other health conditions (e.g., diabetes), while 150 BPM is considered a very fast cadence that might be used with advanced or highly skilled and highly conditioned participants. Nevertheless, recent studies have shown a major increase in the biomechanical load when cadences faster than 135 BPM are used (Santos-Rocha et al. 2006). In aerobics, instructors usually use faster cadences (140 to 170 BPM). If the class includes beginners, elderly people or people from other special populations, instructors must focus their attention on these clients. Knowing about the magnitude of biomechanical and metabolic loading helps instructors select cadences and movements that improve the effectiveness of the activity for health and fitness (Santos-Rocha et al. 2009; Turner and Robling 2003).

Using Music to Motivate Participants

Music is also a very important tool for motivating the participants. The effect of music on mood and vigour during exercise is of particular importance (Hayakawa et al. 2000). Group fitness to music classes involve several forms of exercise that can be performed by a large number of people, regardless of age and fitness level. These two factors (age and fitness level) help determine music selection (high or low BPM) because, for example, elderly, pregnant or obese people move more slowly. Age is also important when choosing rhythm and type of music. Thus, in order to motivate participants, the choice of music is crucial.

Structuring a Group Fitness to Music Class

In order for music to be a helpful tool, fitness instructors need to structure their classes accordingly. When preparing a fitness class, the instructor must select movements or exercises and propose a number of repetitions for each exercise that fits the music structure previously described. Movements used in fitness classes usually need four counts (music beats), or multiples of four. Some exercises need only two beats, but in this case instructors always ask clients to execute an even number of repetitions, ending up using multiples of four beats. The number of repetitions should take into account the music structure just described, meaning that a set of exercises should last 4 beats; 8 beats; 16 beats or multiples of 32 beats.

On the other hand, music also needs to be suited for the specific activity and phase of the class. As mentioned in the previous section, some activities require lower BPM's while others can be practiced with higher BPM's. Likewise, different phases of any class, such as the warm-up, the main activity and the cool-down phase, may also need appropriate music selections and proper structuring.

Warm-Up

In general, the role of the warm-up phase of the class is to prepare the participants' bodies for exercise by making a smooth transition from resting state to exercise. The instructor must select exercises well suited for accomplishing this purpose. The warm-up can also be used to rehearse or introduce movements or routines that will be used in the main part of the class. The cadence may get progressively faster during the warm-up until reaching the intended cadence for the main phase, or main activity, of the class.

Main Activity

The exercises and routines included in the main part of the workout depend on the objectives of the class. The music selected by the instructor must comply with the structure described in the previous section and will set the movement cadence and the rhythm of the movements.

The intensity of the workout can be manipulated by four main factors:

1. **Adjusting the cadence.** The cadence should increase progressively during the session. Instructors must adapt the chosen cadence to the fitness and skill level of the participants.

2. **Adjusting the type of movements included in choreography** (e.g., propulsive movements). Instructors should also adapt the following to the needs of participants: type of movement patterns included in choreography, variations, combinations and progressions. Additionally, participants should master foot movements before adding arm movements.

3. **Adjusting the complexity of choreography** (e.g., complex variations of basic steps and progressions). While some movements are considered basic, others are quite intense, and they might not be recommended for people with certain health conditions (e.g., the use of propulsive movements with pregnant or elderly people).

4. **Adjusting bench height.** Bench height can be adjusted from 10 to 25 centimetres (4 to 10 inches). The 10-centimetre benches are more appropriate for pregnant woman, beginners, elderly people, young people and short people. They can also be used when instructors or participants are tired. Taller or more skilled participants might prefer 20- to 25-centimetre benches. Most participants use benches 15 centimetres tall.

In order to effectively conduct a group fitness class, instructors should select the right type of fitness music and the proper music cadence. They should use music as a tool for counting and setting the rhythm and should perform a proper demonstration of exercises according to the music's rhythm and cadence.

Cool-Down

In general terms, the role of the cool-down phase of the class is to make a smooth transition between exercise and resting state, restore heart rate, and prevent muscle soreness. The instructor must select exercises suitable for accomplishing this objective. Cool-down exercises may either reinforce the movements or routines just performed in the main part of the class or prepare participants for the movements or routines that will be included in future classes. Music for this part may range from electronic dance and pop music during cool-downs to slow relaxing music during stretches.

Basic Moves for a Self-Designed Group Fitness to Music Class

Instructors can combine basic moves and movement patterns to create sequences and choreographies. Fitness movement patterns are defined according to a sequence of steps and touches or elevations (Franco and Santos 1999):

- **Step:** when the participant's foot is placed on the floor and the participant's body weight is transferred to that leg and foot.
- **Touch or elevation:** when the participant does any movement with one leg while bearing the body weight on the other leg and foot (i.e., no transfer of body weight). During the movement, the foot may touch the floor (*touch*) or not (*elevation*).
- **Step plus touch or elevation:** A two-beat movement pattern in which the participant performs a step (beat 1) and then executes a touch or elevation (beat 2) (e.g., step touch).
- **Elevation or touch plus step:** A two-beat movement pattern in which the participant performs a touch or elevation (beat 1) and then performs a step (beat 2) (e.g., touch front).
- **Three steps plus touch or elevation:** A four-beat movement pattern in which the participant performs three steps during the first three beats (one step for each beat) and in the fourth beat performs a touch or elevation (e.g., grapevine).
- **Consecutive alternating steps:** In this one-beat movement pattern, the participant performs a step on every beat, alternating between the right and left legs at all times (e.g., marching).
- **Consecutive simultaneous steps:** In this one-beat movement pattern, the participant performs steps with both legs simultaneously in every beat (e.g., jumping jacks).

A step aerobics class contains the following movement patterns (Franco and Santos 1999):

- **Step plus touch or elevation in the 2nd beat:** Participant steps up on the bench on the 1st, 3rd and 4th beats and performs a touch or elevation in the 2nd beat (e.g., alternating knee lift, leg curl, or step touch).
- **Step plus touch or elevation in the 4th beat:** Participant steps up on the bench on the 1st, 2nd and 3rd beats and performs a touch or elevation on the 4th beat on or above the floor (e.g., over the top or across the top).

- **Step plus touch or elevation in the 2nd and 4th beats:** Participant steps up on the bench on the 1st and 3rd beats and performs a touch or elevation on the bench on the 2nd beat and on the floor on the 4th beat (e.g., step touch up and down, L-step).

- **Consecutive alternating steps without touches or elevations:** Participant performs steps alternating between right and left feet (e.g., basic step, V-step).

- **Consecutive simultaneous steps without touches or elevations:** Participant moves both feet at the same time (e.g., twist step, skip, jumps). Steps may alternate direction of movement.

Leading Movement and the Leading Leg

The leading of any movement can be classified according to its laterality and nature. The leading of a movement depends on the leg that starts the movement, which determines the leading laterality. The leading leg is the one that begins the movement, followed by the impulsion or trail leg. Sometimes both legs start the movement. When analysing the laterality of any movement or step, identify which leg is leading. The laterality of a movement can be defined as *right leading* or *left leading* (e.g., basic step, march, knee lift, grapevine) as well as *neutral*, where both legs lead simultaneously (e.g., jump, twist, jumping jacks).

Another important thing to consider is the nature of the leading movement. The leading nature of any movement is determined by both the leg that starts the movement and the leg that is naturally positioned, at the end of that same movement, to perform the next movement. When the step that follows a leading movement is performed with the same leading leg, it is called a *simple leading movement* (e.g., basic step, V-step, march, jog). When the step that follows the leading movement is performed with the other leg (the opposite of the one that led the first movement), it is called an *alternating leading movement* (e.g., knee lift, over the top, grapevine). When a movement is performed with both legs or feet at the same time (e.g., jump, twist or jumping jack), it is called *neutral leading*. The leading nature of a movement is determined according to the number of steps contained within one movement, irrespective of the number of touches or elevations. A paired number of steps results in simple leading and an odd number of steps results in alternating leading.

As with single moments, instructors should understand the leading nature of an exercise routine or choreography when planning and teaching group fitness classes to music. They must balance mechanical loading between the two legs to prevent fatigue and long-term injuries. In the case of choreography, as defined by a set of movements, the number of alternating and simple leading movements within a piece of choreography will determine its leading nature. A paired or even number of alternating leading movements will result in a simple leading choreography, and an odd number of alternating leading movements will result in an alternating leading choreography. Instructors can include as many alternating leading movements as they want, but they must include the same number of repetitions for both the right and left legs. For alternating leading movements any paired number of repetitions will ensure a proper balance between right and left executions. However, special care must be taken when considering simple leading movements. For instance, simple leading movements do not allow for balanced leg work (same number of repetitions with both legs) in an exercise routine, especially in step aerobics, unless they are combined with alternating leading movements.

This means that when planning class choreography, instructors must consider the type of movements (or similar moves in terms of leading leg), the number of repetitions on each side and the links between them. They should be aware that any change in leading leg for a movement will completely change the choreography.

Knowing the characteristics of and differences among neutral, simple and alternating movement leading enables instructors to make smooth transitions between exercises. This is of particular importance when considering a musical eight or a musical phrase. Instructors should be aware that ending a musical eight or a musical phrase with a neutral leading move can confuse participants, since it is not always clear after a neutral leading move which leg should lead next.

They should also consider the best use of exercises in different movement planes and whether available classroom space can accommodate directional changes in the choreography.

Verbally and Visually Cueing an Exercise Routine

To help participants properly follow the exercise routines, instructors must have clear, effective and specific communication skills. These communication skills might be related to different purposes: to give an instruction or command to perform an exercise, to provide feed-back on the performance of an exercise or, simply, to motivate the clients. Good communication between the instructor and the clients is essential for delivering an effective class workout. Instructors may use the following techniques:

- **Verbal/auditory:** The instructor uses verbal communication and the participants listen.
- **Gestural/visual:** The instructor uses gestures to communicate while the participants watch.

Instructors may use a combination of the two to complement one another. In these communication methods, instructors can use at least three main forms of instructions or commands for the partic-ipants to follow. These commands are characterised by the timed sequence of movements (choreography) and music:

- **Descriptive:** The instructor explains the move the participants are supposed to perform before the movement occurs in the sequence. The time required for giving a descriptive command depends on the amount of information the instructor wants to relate. This instruction ends when another command is needed.
- **Regressive:** The instructor informs the participants how much time they have before changing movement, sequence, direc-tion, plane of movement and so on. When giving a regressive command instructors must allow participants ample time to prepare for the next move. Usually, instructors count down the four steps before the new movement, giving a verbal cue on each beat of the last four moves ('New move in 4, 3, 2 and 1'; see figure 8.4).
- **Pre-emptive (forward looking):** The instructor uses this com-mand immediately before beginning the next move, usually during the last two beats. Instructors should clearly call out a short, recognisable word such as the name of the step (e.g., 'Basic step!' or 'Grapevine!') or an action (e.g., 'clap', 'go', 'kick!' or 'jump!'). This command is the last information participants receive before making the next move (figure 8.5).

In addition to giving commands, in order to effectively reach all the participants, instructors must take care to project their voices from several teaching points in the room. They should also provide demonstrations from several angles and positions throughout the room.

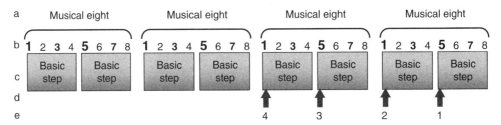

Figure 8.4 Scheme of a regressive command during the last four moves. (a) music structure; (b) downbeats and on-beats (bold) and upbeats; (c) exercises or choreography; (d) command timing; (e) command content.

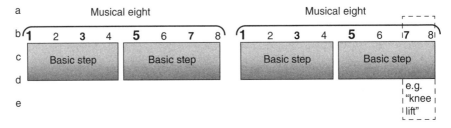

Figure 8.5 Scheme of a pre-emptive command during the last two counts. (a) music structure; (b) downbeats and on-beats (bold) and upbeats; (c) exercises or choreography; (d) command content; (e) (dotted line) command timing.

Conclusion

Bottom line, the instructor's job is incredibly challenging. It requires a strong body of knowledge that is multidisciplinary as well as trained skills and competencies to ensure safe, joyful and successful classes. The challenge new fitness instructors face can be overcome by learning, preparation and training. In this chapter, we focused on the basic knowledge and skills for preparing and leading fitness group classes to music. Mastering these contents will provide strong tools and empower fitness instructors to achieve high standards of success in leading fitness group classes to music.

Music and Choreography

Lenka Velínská

Music in dynamic group classes (e.g., aerobics, dance aerobics, step, total body workout or body styling) is not just a mere background, but a fundamental element that influences the entire class. Harmony between the exercise and the music is implied. Instructors must respect not only the rhythm and tempo of music but also its regular structure in phrases and blocks. Instructors of group aerobics classes must be able to synchronise the exercise with the music and lead the group of participants through the musical routine. To do this, they must understand musical structure and feel confident working with it, easily recognising the beginnings of blocks and phrases.

Accurate use of music helps instructors maintain the appropriate intensity of movements and, accordingly, meet the goals of aerobic or fitness training. Music is also a very important motivator, allowing instructors to work at various energy levels and build up positive atmosphere in the class by adapting the tempo, rhythm and type of music to match participant preferences.

Musical Tempo

Tempo—the speed or pace of music—is related to movement cadence. This aspect of music helps instructors maintain appropriate exercise intensity. An exercise pace that is too slow does not enable the heart rate to rise into the training zone; a pace that is too fast impairs the performance technique of individual movements and takes the exercise intensity all the way to the anaerobic zone, which is not suitable for group training because the benefits of aerobic exercise disappear.

The tempo or speed of a piece is indicated in BPM (beats per minute), and every type of group fitness to music class, as well as individual segments of the class, has given reference BPM values (table 9.1). Of course, these intervals might be adapted according to the level of fitness and skills of the participants.

Musical Structure

Music designated for group fitness classes has a regular form. The following terms are useful when describing its structure (table 9.2).

With group fitness classes, instructors use music composed of regularly repeated blocks of 32 beats. Each section leads into the next without pause, without any irregularities (missing beats or extra beats). By using *phrased music*, instructors achieve maximum continuity of movements and trouble-free harmony between the music and the exercise (table 9.3).

As previously mentioned the musical structure and its division into phrases and blocks serve as the cornerstone for the structure of the whole class. Every exercise is performed to a particular number of beats. Table 9.4 shows some examples of moves and steps according to the number of beats (2, 4 and 8).

Table 9.1 Terms Used to Describe Music Structure

Beat	The basic unit of time in music structure
Downbeat	Accented, strong beat
Upbeat	Unaccented, weak beat
Phrase	Measure of 8 counts, 1st count of the phrase is more accentuated than others
Block	Collection of four 8-count measures (i.e., 32 counts)
Master downbeat	1st count of a block; audibly the strongest count of musical structure

Table 9.2 The 32 Beats Included in a Musical Block

1st phrase	1	2	3	4	5	6	7	8
2nd phrase	1	2	3	4	5	6	7	8
3rd phrase	1	2	3	4	5	6	7	8
4th phrase	1	2	3	4	5	6	7	8

Table 9.3   Reference Intervals of Beats per Minute (BPM) for Different Types of Group Fitness to Music Classes

Type of class (examples)	BPM reference interval
Aerobics, aerobic dance, power aerobics	135–145 BPM
Body styling, total body workout	133–138 BPM
Step aerobics, power step	130–134 BPM
Core training, Bosu	120–130 BPM
MTV dance, house dance	100–130 BPM

Table 9.4   Examples of Moves and Steps According to the Number of Beats (2, 4 and 8)

Number of beats	Sample moves and steps
2	Tap, cha-cha, step touch, leg curl, knee in, march (walking), half mambo
4	Mambo, V-step, reverse V-step, grapevine, cross march, pivot turn
8	March (forward and backward), L-step, box step

Cross Phrase

Cross phrase, a term that began in the mid-1990s, is an intentional breach of the regular musical phrase for higher variability of steps. By programming steps to irregular numbers of beats (2, 4, 8, 16 or 32 beats), instructors can introduce new steps and combination options. In the context of music for group lessons, instructors frequently use a cross phrase within a block of 8 or 16 beats. However, the contemporary trend of asymmetric dance choreography is leading instructors to introduce cross phrases within larger units of 32 or even 64 beats. Cross phrases can be challenging because the musical lead is discontinued. Also, instructors must be very confident and precise in their performance of the new pattern, and must carefully prepare a methodical approach for progressively teaching the transition.

In contrast with the terminology for the majority of all other phrases and steps, the definitions of cross phrases and their steps are not universal. Thus instructors may come across varied names for the same step or cross phrase variations with the same name as the original phrase. Table 9.5 shows some examples of moves and steps according to the number of beats (3, 5, 6 and 7).

No-Tap Choreography

Steps used in group fitness to music classes are classified according to the number of musical beats they use and their characteristics from the viewpoint of how they combine with other steps.

When linking the steps and creating blocks of movement, many instructors use no-tap choreography. In the context of fitness and dance, a *tap* occurs when you touch a foot to the ground without transferring the body's weight to that side (e.g., step touch). No-tap choreography continually alternates the leading leg between the right and left sides, drawing inspiration from walking, the most natural human motion. This creates maximum ease during the transition between steps and continuity of movement, which helps keep heart rate in the aerobic zone. Table 9.6 shows the characteristics and some examples of the different groups of steps that work well with no-tap choreography.

Table 9.5   Examples of Moves and Steps According to the Number of Beats (3, 5, 6 and 7)

Number of beats	Sample moves and steps
3	Stomp (baby mambo, rock), salsa (tango)
5	Double stomp (double baby mambo, double rock)
6	Repeater 2
7	Triple stomp (triple baby mambo, triple rock)

Table 9.6   Steps Compatible with No-Tap Choreography

Group of steps	Characteristics	Samples
1. Nonalternating steps	Leading leg stays constant: After performing a nonalternating step starting on the right side, the right leg naturally leads again on the accented (strong) beat of the music. Should instructors wish to lead next with left leg instead, they would have to add a tap.	Marching or walking V-step Basic Reverse V-step Mambo
2. Alternating steps	Leading leg alternates sides: After performing an alternating step leading with the right side, the left side naturally leads on the accented (strong) beat of the music, and vice versa. Should instructors wish to keep continuing with the same leading leg, they would have to add a tap.	Step touch Step knee up Tap Grapevine Cha-cha-cha Plié or lunge
3. Neutral steps	Neutral steps end in the basic stand, from which either the right or left side could lead. These steps should be integrated in choreographic classes infrequently, particularly at the end of the blocks, because at the end of the movement, it is unclear to students which side should lead next.	Jumping jack Squat

The no-tap principle makes it clear which leg should lead next, which keeps participants from stopping or concentrating on foot movement to the detriment of correct technique or posture. Since instructors, in turn, do not have to keep announcing which foot or side should lead, they can pay more attention to giving feedback.

Having learned musical structure and step characteristics, instructors can next build the lesson's choreography by using the no-tap principle to combine individual exercises into blocks of 32 counts and then join these blocks into a routine. Table 9.7 presents several alternating and nonalternating steps according to the number of beats.

Choreography

For more than 20 years, instructors of group fitness to music classes have been combining individual exercises and steps into blocks and then linking blocks to form choreography. Choreography is understood as an assemblage of several (mostly two to five) 32-count blocks, but instructors may also work with 16-count blocks. Instructors primarily use choreography to form the main part of aerobic lessons because repeating familiar steps in new combinations keeps participants' heart rates in the training zone. Additional benefits of choreography include practicing the correct technique of movements

Table 9.7 Examples of Alternating and Nonalternating Steps and Step Sequences According to the Number of Beats

Beats	Alternating steps	Nonalternating steps
2	Tap Step touch Side to side Leg curl Cha-cha-cha Lunge	March Half mambo
4	Step tap, kick, knee lift Double side to side, leg curl, knee in Grapevine Mambo cha-cha Plié Travel side to side, kick, knee	March, open march Straddle V-step, reverse V-step, basic step Mambo, pivot
8	Repeater tap, kick, knee lift Single, single, double knee, curl L-step	Any combination of previous nonalternating step examples totalling 8 beats

(instructors repeat each step in different combinations; therefore participants have the opportunity to continually perfect their technique without getting bored), increasing motivation, and developing muscle memory, co-ordination and kinetic orientation. Every lesson has a particular objective.

Instructors may use two types of choreography:

- **Symmetric choreography** contains one alternating step (both right and left leading), and the entire block is performed on both sides equally. This choreography is employed particularly in build-up and shape-up types of aerobic lessons and in step aerobics.

- **Asymmetric choreography** contains an even number of alternating steps. The choreography is partially performed on the right side and partially on the left, but the parts are not identical. This type of choreography is often applied in dance lessons.

Tables 9.8 and 9.9 present examples of a symmetric block and an asymmetric block, respectively.

In practice, and particularly in dance choreography, instructors may come up with combinations of symmetric and asymmetric parts or may alternate 32-count blocks with combinations of 16-count blocks. It is all a matter of the instructor's creativity and experience. However, the outcome is essential: The choreography must correspond with the musical structure by filling several (usually three to five) musical blocks of 32 counts (table 9.10).

Table 9.8   Sample of Symmetric Block: 1 × 32 Counts to the Right + 1 × 32 Counts to the Left

Beats	Move	Direction	Variations	Leading foot
8	Step kick (×2)	Forward	Knee up	R/L
8	Repeater step kick	Forward	Step kick, twist back and forth, step kick	R
8	March + 1/2 mambo (×2)	Forward / backward	Spin back	L
8	V + reverse V-step		Basic + reverse basic or 2 basic steps	L
8	Step kick (×2)	Forward		L/R
8	Repeater step kick	Forward	Step kick, twist back and forth, step kick	L
8	March + 1/2 mambo (×2)	Forward / backward	Spin back	R
8	V + reverse V-step			R

Table 9.9 **Sample of Asymmetric Block: 1 × 32 Counts to the Right or Left**

Beats	Move	Direction	Variations	Leading foot
8	Step kick (×2)	Forward		R/L
8	Repeater step kick	Forward	Step kick, twist back and forth, step kick	R
4	Mambo cha-cha-cha	Forward / backward	Cha-cha 180° turn	L
4	1/2 pivot + march	Forward / backward		R
8	V + reverse V-step			R

Table 9.10 **Sample of Structure of Combined Choreography: 4 × 32 Counts**

Structure	Choreography	Music
1st block	Symmetric block of 16 counts R; 16 counts L	32 beats
2nd block	Asymmetric block	32 beats
3rd block	Symmetric block of 32 counts R	32 beats
4th block	Symmetric block of 32 counts L	32 beats

Whether instructors decide to use symmetric or asymmetric choreography or a combination thereof, they must bear in mind that choreography is not the objective of the lesson, but a tool that helps them teach the lesson's objective in an interesting and enjoyable manner.

The lessons' objective always consists primarily of aerobic training that is beneficial to health. Therefore, choreography should meet the following requirements:

- Choreography must correspond to the clients' proficiency level. If the group members have diverse skill levels, which is often the case in fitness centres, instructors must prepare choreography to accommodate various difficulty levels.

- Choreography must be continuous. Steps, transitions and blocks should naturally join one another. They should take advantage of gravitational pull and the natural direction of movement, which allows movements to be easily repeated. Instructors should use the no-tap principle so that participants have only one option when choosing a leading leg.

- Choreography should be balanced in several aspects:
  - **Equal use of right and left legs.** In symmetric choreography and with proper teaching procedures, this is a given, but even asymmetric choreography can strain the right and left legs in a balanced although not entirely identical way, if it is set up and taught well.
  - **Directional balance.** Choreography should employ and combine movements in various directions, not just to the right and left or forwards and backwards, as is often the habit. Instructors may use diagonal directions as well as varied forms (e.g., square, triangle or circle). Movement in space increases the exercise intensity even without using high-impact steps (based on jumps and running). It develops co-ordination and spatial orientation and enables the instructor to keep creating new combinations from familiar steps.
  - **Intensity.** Choreography alternate less intensive steps (e.g., low-impact moves on the spot) with very intensive steps (e.g., high-impact moves with large spatial shift). Instructors should increase intensity towards the end of the main part of the session.
  - **Arm work.** In balanced choreography, the arm work complements the leg work. Of course, participants should master leg and foot movements before adding arm work. Instructors should engage the arms reasonably since arm work escalates the exercise intensity. Instructors should not use complicated arm movements in moments of sophisticated co-ordination. They should also watch out for participants who push their arms forward, which places inappropriate overload on deltoid muscles and contributes to incorrect use of the upper part of the trapezius muscle.
- Choreography should be well arranged and clear. Instructors should try not to incorporate identical steps, at least not at the beginning and the end of blocks. They can help orient participants by naming the blocks (e.g., according to their form or first or somehow significant move).
- Choreography must comply with criteria for injury prevention and should be suitable for the general public.
- Choreography should be interesting, fun and motivating. It should carry the participants away.

Conclusion

The instructor's awareness of music is a vital part of a group fitness class. Music is a working tool for the instructor, because music determines the movement speed and can act as a stimulant, which can increase performance, respiration and cardiac rate. Not only can music help intensify the workout by reducing the factors that contribute to pain, tension, anxiety and discomfort, but music also can provide guidance to the instructor in terms of counting the number of repetitions of an exercise or a choreographic sequence. Besides motivating, music makes the movement experience enjoyable and gives more time for the instructor to provide feedback. Therefore it's important that instructors create a choreography routine using the correct rhythm and musical structure, keeping in mind the movement pattern and intensity of the exercises along with the client's level of performance. After mastering the points presented in this chapter, instructors will be ready to choose class music and prepare appropriate choreography.

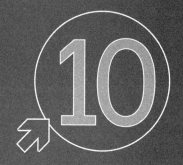

Ending a Session

Jana Havrdová
Nuno Pimenta

After reviewing the points presented in chapters 6 through 9, instructors will be ready to end the session properly. The end of a class should be a moment of joy, when the participants can congratulate themselves for their achievements and feel good about themselves for being active, for being able to be active and for accomplishing one more enjoyable class. This is a moment of the class when instructors will want to make their clients feel particularly good about what they have done in the class and everything that they have accomplished and, subsequently, feel eager to come back for the next class. This contradicts the idea that the ending of a class is just the conclusion of an exercise or training unit where people cool down and stretch. In fact it can and should be much more than that. Little has been researched and written about this topic, and most knowledge on the subject comes from experience in gyms and competitive clubs.

The end of a class is the perfect opportunity for instructors to both give important feedback to the clients and receive feedback from them. When giving feedback to clients, instructors should focus on the following:

- Praising beginners or new clients
- Highlighting clients who did particularly well (clients who revealed great commitment to the class goals) or pointing out desirable behaviours

- Encouraging and giving positive feedback to those who seemed less focused or unmotivated or who made a lot of mistakes during the class
- Inviting clients to the next class or to a follow-up class of a different type of exercise, or to participate in other events organised either by the instructor or the club
- Increasing self-efficacy and boosting adherence (see the behavioural theories in the section 'The Instructor's Role')
- Making announcements about special occasions, including club holidays or special events
- Acknowledging aspects of clients' private lives so that their peers can encourage them at the end of class (e.g., singing birthday songs, applauding any public professional or personal achievement) and help them feel they are part of a family (Note: this may be discouraged by club policy.)

As just mentioned, the end of a class is also a time for receiving feedback from the clients. Feedback from the clients may include the following:

- General opinion on how the class went
- Likes and dislikes about the class
- How they felt during exercise

Instructors should be good listeners, and they should make themselves available to their clients. This time can help them gather important information and feedback that may have significant implications for planning and organising their classes and exercise sessions.

Occasionally, for scheduling reasons, clients have to leave class before the end. Instructors should be open to this, but they should also inform clients in advance about the importance of the end of the class. By having the clients stay until the very end of a class, in addition to properly addressing the major goals of cooling down, stretching and relaxing, the instructor gains extra space to communicate further and motivate the clients to commit to regular exercise. The end of a class is also used for clearing away exercise equipment and materials used in the class. Clients should be encouraged to do this together as a team-building exercise, which facilitates personal bonds among participants.

From a more intentional and technical perspective, the end of a class may be regarded from two different points of view:

- Interest in and need for communication on the part of **the instructor**
- Interest in and need for communication on the part of **the club**

The Instructor's Role

Fitness instructors need to understand that clients are their real bosses. They are the ones who are paying the checks. Without clients, there would be no classes for fitness instructors to lead. This sets the tone for the attention that any fitness instructor should give to every part of the class that involves clients. One key aspect of the fitness instructor interaction with the clients, which is the dominant feature of the end of a fitness class, is communication proficiency. Instructors of fitness classes must have within themselves the tools to assure professional, correct, joyful and powerful communication. This is true for communication with anyone in the club, from the club manager to other instructors and, particularly, the clients.

At the end of a class, instructors should establish meaningful communication with clients. Some instructors struggle to connect with clients in a less formal and unstructured fashion. This happens particularly with instructors new to teaching fitness classes who are focusing their communication skills on describing the exercises and movements well (Bonelli 2000). When novice instructors gain experience, the communication about exercises will become second nature to them and they can start communicating with clients about motivational aspects of the class and creating an environment where clients feel good about the class and themselves (Bonelli 2000). Some instructors, however, struggle more than others when it comes to interpersonal communication. Certain personalities may constrain their capacity to interact with others and, therefore, may jeopardise their communication skills. Introverts will likely face significantly greater challenges in establishing personal contact with clients than extroverts will. Regardless of their personality type, instructors can work to reach a high standard of interpersonal communication. Instructors who need to work on enhancing their communication skills can use the following strategy, which will help them improve with practice:

- Outside of class, instructors can come up with short phrases that they think will be nice and important to use at the end of a class (e.g., 'I'm very proud of you', 'You were heroes today', 'Great job', 'That's what I'm talking about' and so on).

- Instructors should practise saying these phrases, in front of a mirror if necessary, and try to find the best way to look and sound convincing.

After having found specific authentic sentences that clients would like to hear at the end of a class and practised them aloud to reach a natural way of saying them convincingly, instructors will be ready to apply these trained communication techniques in real classes.

Because they believe the messages, feel comfortable transmitting those feelings and can now convey them in a convincing way as a result of the training, even shy or introverted instructors can overcome their difficulties and ensure professional competence and successful communication with clients. Instructors who put in the time and effort to practise will attain high levels of proficiency in communicating with the clients.

Instructors must hone their social skills when addressing clients. They should be capable of correctly assessing privacy boundaries and sensing what clients are willing to share. In most cases it is a good thing to learn the names of all clients and address them by their names. This usually makes the clients feel good and important because they are recognised as individuals rather than as just another participant. Some clients have specific preferences that instructors should be ready to accommodate, such as the wish to be addressed in terms of their professional or political position (e.g., engineer or senator) or even their academic degree (e.g., doctor or professor). Instructors should not let this type of wish get in the way of setting significant and lasting bonds with their clients. The better and the more agreeable the instructor–client relations are, the greater the effect the instructor will have on the physical and mental condition of the client and the longer their professional relationship will last. The instructor should also focus on the clients' attitude towards exercise. In order to address this concern, the instructor should be equipped with behavioural tools based on theories and models that aim to enhance exercise adherence and maintenance.

Several theories and models have been proposed that may be useful in supporting behavioural interventions for fitness instructors and increasing recreational physical activity (ACSM 2013). These include the theory of self-efficacy, the self-determination theory and the transtheoretical model (ACSM 2013).

Self-efficacy has been defined as one's belief in his or her capabilities to organise and execute the courses of action required to achieve a given goal (Ashford et al. 2010). The concept of self-efficacy relies on the postulate that 'cognitive processes mediate behaviour change but that cognitive events are induced and altered more readily by experience of mastery arising from effective performance' (Bandura 1977, p. 191). According to this theoretical framework, instructors may promote exercise participation or adherence by increasing clients' awareness or belief that they are capable of completing the tasks proposed in class (Ashford et al. 2010). Self-efficacy is the central component of many behavioural theories (Ashford et al. 2010).

The transtheoretical model, initially proposed by Prochaska and colleagues (1992) to help change addictive behaviours, has been adapted to help people adopt exercise behaviours (Hutchison et al. 2009). According to this theory everyone is considered to be in one of five proposed stages of readiness for behavioural changes (Hutchison et al. 2009). Since they have already taken the first step by signing up for the class, all clients should be in one of the three more advanced stages of readiness for behavioural change: preparation (intending to be regularly active in the next 30 days or already somewhat active but not meeting yet the minimal physical activity recommendations), action (regularly active for less than 6 months) or maintenance (regularly active for 6 months or more) (Spencer et al. 2006). The feedback instructors offer clients in the preparation stage differs from that given to clients in the action and maintenance stages.

Ultimately, the instructor's challenge is to make sure that every client moves to the maintenance stage and stays there. For that, instructors can benefit from strategies on the variables involved in planning classes and exercise sessions and making adjustments for particular clients. In terms of the ending of class sessions, the transtheoretical model has the most influence on instructors' communication with clients, depending on what stage of readiness for behavioural change the client is in. As mentioned, self-efficacy has an important role in the client's transition to the action or maintenance stages (Spencer et al. 2006).

Another keystone concept is the self-determination theory (ACSM 2013). This theory focuses on motivation, distinguishing among amotivation (lack of intention to engage in exercise), extrinsic motivation (engaging in exercise for reasons dissociated from the behaviour itself, e.g., 'I exercise because I want to lose weight') and intrinsic motivation (engaging in exercise for pure joy and satisfaction associated to the behaviour itself, e.g., 'I exercise because I love it!') (Silva et al. 2008). This theory also distinguishes between self-determined (resulting from the client's own choice and volition, e.g., 'I decided to participate in exercise and my goal is...') and controlled motivation (resulting from pressure from others rather from the clients themselves, e.g., 'My doctor told me to start exercising.') (Silva et al. 2008). Apparently when people engage in a behaviour, such as exercise, as a result of a self-determined motivation and then associate that behaviour with enjoyment and satisfaction, they are more likely to sustain it in the long run (Teixeira et al. 2012).

In other words, according to the theory of self-determination, the instructor's challenge is to plan and adapt the routines and communicate with clients in order to transform exercise into an enjoyable and satisfactory experience. As much as possible, instructors should also help clients locate their own motivation to exercise. Communication with clients at the end of a class may facilitate this goal. In order to engage in more intentional and proficient communication with clients, particularly at the end of classes, fitness instructors should work on communication techniques in accordance with the framework established in effective behavioural theories. This approach may enhance the instructors' skills in communicating and promoting exercise adherence. Sound introductory publications in the field of behavioural change regarding exercise are widely available (ACSM 2013; Napolitano 2013; Martin 2013; McClanahan 2013). This chapter makes only a brief mention of theoretical approaches to fundamental behavioural change. Instructors interested in strengthening their knowledge and competency in this field should look for additional resources.

As mentioned earlier, the end of a class is also an opportunity for instructors to gather important feedback from the clients about the class. This, along with the instructors' own thoughts about the participants' strengths and areas for growth, should allow for the most important part of the class: reflection. After every class, the instructor should engage participants in a time of reflection about everything that just happened in the class. These approaches and techniques will help fitness instructors enhance their competence and become better fitness professionals, which can also ensure that their work will provide a steady source of income. Fitness instructors may apply these new competencies in a wide number of professional settings. Reflection applies not only to regular classes, but also to short- or long-term workshops and active holidays with exercise. Caring for clients after class plays a major role in building up business relationships between both parties.

The Club's Role

From the perspective of the owner or group fitness manager, the instructor's performance at the end of class is clearly important, both for operational and commercial reasons. The operational requirements are absolutely clear-cut. A class taking place within a scheduled time bracket needs to start and end on time. Before clients start to arrive for the next class, all equipment must be cleared away, and all participants from the previous class must leave. The arrival and departure of clients to and from the training gym must be organised in a manner that prevents difficulties, bottlenecks or bodily harm. In principle, handing the training premises over to the next instructor in good condition sets the next class up for success. The commercial reasons for ending a class well are also obvious—a high-quality conclusion makes clients return to the club and maybe even bring their friends and acquaintances along. Accordingly, good managers should establish the general terms and conditions for ending classes and supervise instructors. Such a model, which is highly effective in practice, may also include an explicit and detailed arrangement of instructor–client communication at the end of class. Instructors may be encouraged to do the following:

- Thank participants for attending the class
- Issue an invitation to next class, stating its date, time and style
- Encourage clients, provide feedback, follow up on any contradictions or ambiguities they sensed from participants during the class and give advice on any negative physical symptoms or sensations that clients might experience in the following days
- Provide information about club events or news (discounts, new schedule, new locations, new training styles)
- Give clear directions for stowing away any equipment and leaving the gym

Accurate and active communication between the manager and the instructors is a key factor for providing successful group classes in a club setting. Instructors perform best when they are satisfied, well informed and motivated.

For a number of clients, the instructor is one of the few club representatives they meet during their visits there. In many countries, clients and instructors form distinctive personal bonds. Often, clients follow their instructors from club to club, seeking their services regardless of place and terms or conditions. Some clubs try to avoid this dependence on instructors. To that end, they establish rigid scripts that instructors must follow when addressing any client, including at the end of classes. This will make staff interventions uniform, leading clients to feel good and well regarded in the club, regardless of which instructor they interact with. A set routine also reduces the odds that strong client–instructor bonds will develop at the club. Underestimating the instructor's drag on clients and giving significant preference to environment may result in substantial reduction in the number of clients attending both group and individual classes.

Conclusion

The bottom line is that the end of class is an extremely important moment for quality results, both for the client and for the fitness club's management, and it must not be underestimated or neglected.

Good preparation on behalf of instructors, including education, planning and training, particularly around everything connected with communication with clients, will determine their proficiency and success. Club managers should accurately set up the terms and conditions of instructor intervention and attitudes. Doing so will lead to positive effects and organisational success.

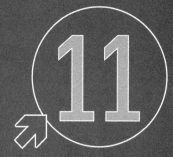

Safety Guidelines for Group Fitness to Music

Susana Moral González
Sonia García Merino

This chapter describes the basic safety requirements that instructors should consider before starting a group fitness class. If they take into account all of these essential aspects during the planning stage, their classes will successfully avoid unnecessary risks. This chapter provides instructors with information about their legal and insurance responsibilities with respect to the national guidelines, recommended alternatives and modifications for use when planning a class activity, health and safety checks related to the exercise environment and appropriate responses to a medical emergency.

Legal and Insurance Responsibilities

With respect to national guidelines, group fitness instructors have a number of duties and responsibilities connected with their service to clients. Some standards are specific to instructors, and others apply for fitness centres (Connaughton 1998). Failure to comply with the standards of practice can cause problems with the law, but adherence helps minimise legal issues.

Standards of Practice for Group Fitness Instructors

■ If fitness facilities do screen new clients (using procedures such as the PAR-Q or a Health/Fitness Facility Preparticipation Screening Questionnaire) to assess whether they can safely execute an exercise programme, instructors must apply the appropriate protocols themselves to detect possible risks before allowing participants to start the programme or activity.

■ Testing the client's fitness level and programming the activity are essential tasks for group fitness instructors. Component fitness evaluations allow instructors to tailor the programme or activity to the fitness level of the participants and to monitor progress. They should pay attention to the intensity, frequency, type and duration of the exercise in their programmes, modifying and adapting these aspects as needed over time. Group fitness instructors must ensure that the class activity is appropriate to the participants' level of fitness.

■ Group fitness instructors should check to see whether clients are performing the different exercises properly, correcting those who need help and modifying exercises to meet the needs of the participants.

■ Instructors must regularly inspect classroom equipment and log the results of their inspection. Any damaged equipment should be promptly repaired to prevent an accident.

■ Instructors who adhere to the standards of practice minimise risk during fitness activities. In an emergency situation instructors should follow the steps of the facility's emergency plan (for more information, see the section 'Responding Appropriately to a Medical Emergency').

Standards of Practice for Facilities

■ Implement a medical emergency plan supported by qualified personnel.

■ Conduct a health assessment for all new clients before they start class to identify those who might be at risk and modify programmes for people with special needs.

■ Employ professionals who are certified and qualified to properly supervise exercise programmes.

■ Signal areas that may pose a risk.

■ Provide services or programmes for young people who need special care and provide proper supervision at all times.

■ Comply with basic standards for safety, taking into account issues related to lighting, grounds, accessibility and so on.

- Comply with all relevant laws, regulations and published standards.

Facilities that meet these standards of practice usually protect their employees from trouble with the law if an accident occurs during a fitness class. However, this protection does not relieve instructors of their professional responsibilities and duties.

Most of the lawsuits against exercise professionals are due to negligence, which is defined as 'failure to conform one's conduct to a generally accepted standard or duty, which proximately causes harm to an individual to whom the former owed some duty or responsibility' (Herbert 1996). Some of the defences for negligent actions are as follows (McCann 1998):

- **Comparative negligence.** 'Comparative negligence applies when the plaintiff has also been negligent in the case and his or her negligence has contributed to the injury.'

- **Assumption of the risk.** 'In some cases assumption of the risk could be a defence to a negligence claim. There are forms that express assumption of risk by participants.'

- **No negligence.** 'The primary defence could be that your program is not negligent and that the instructors or the equipment checkers acted reasonably and prudently under the circumstances.'

- **Waivers.** 'The use of the waiver while generally not an absolute bar to liability, can often be used effectively to demonstrate that a plaintiff knowingly undertook the risks of the activity. It is worthwhile to have waivers so that they can be used in evidence against the person bringing the claim.'

- **Failure to minimise damages.** 'There is a defence known as failure to minimize damages which means that a plaintiff may not recover to the extent that any injuries he or she received were aggravated by a failure to minimize damages such as by seeking adequate medical care or failing to follow medical advice.'

Planning Class Activity

Teaching a group fitness class should not be spontaneous. Many guidelines offer instructors valuable information about how to teach and plan a group fitness class, as well as how to adapt plans to meet class needs.

The purpose of this section is to help instructors understand their options and how to apply them when preparing for class, as well as what to keep in mind while teaching.

Participants' Needs

The most important thing to consider when preparing for a group fitness class is to design a clear plan of fitness-related activities that fit the needs of a specific group of participants. Taking into account the particular needs and interests of their participants, instructors should work to successfully integrate the exercise principles and behavioural techniques that will motivate clients to participate in sessions and achieve their goals. Many group fitness participants have different levels of fitness and skills, which can pose a big challenge for fitness instructors. Instructors should know the health history and fitness level of each participant in order to appropriately modify the plan or programme if needed.

Preparation

To ensure that they include a variety of exercises in their programmes, use class time efficiently and progress smoothly through their activities, instructors must prepare their classes in advance. When planning, fitness instructors should keep the following in mind:

- Type of exercise or group fitness activity (e.g., aerobics, strength)
- Intensity, duration and frequency of the activity or exercise session
- Specific exercises and how they will be connected
- Music: cadence (BPM) and rhythm
- Necessary equipment
- Class organisation
- Precautions
- Participant feedback

Exercise Selection

When selecting which exercises are best for a particular class, instructors should consider the characteristics of the participants and their goals. Knowledge about human anatomy and biomechanics, as well as about the factors that affect efficient human movement, is really important for fitness instructors. When selecting exercises, instructors must choose carefully. In class, they should first demonstrate every single exercise to the participants, showing them the correct technique. They should remember to give participants feedback on their technique during the exercise, since not all participants will know how to do the exercise correctly. Of course, the chosen exercises must always be effective and safe for the participants.

Supplementary Equipment

If instructors are going to use any kind of equipment in the class, they should prepare it in advance so participants can easily access it when the time comes. They should explain when and how participants should use the equipment. Participants who attend more frequently may decide on their own when to use equipment (if the instructor has previously shown them how to use it). In this case, participants can put away their equipment when the class is finished.

Class Organisation

Everyone in a group fitness class should be able to hear the instructions and see the instructor's demonstrations. Instructors must organise the class to ensure that all participants have equal advantages. In classes where the instructor stands in front of the class, the participants who have the best motor skills tend to take the first few rows, while the participants who have less experience stand in the back. Because of this, instructors must move around the room, giving all participants the opportunity to be in the first row at least once. Of course, instructors have different teaching strategies, and they will decide each time which teaching approach will be the most effective that day for helping participants properly learn the exercises and movements.

   When the instructors themselves have less professional experience, preparing and programming the class requires extra work and time. After getting some experience, these procedures will become easier.

Health and Safety Checks

When the class starts, instructors should be sure that the environment is safe for the participants and it is ready for the activity that is about to start. Instructors must ensure that equipment is in good condition. Instructors should keep the following tips in mind:

- All equipment must be serviced on a regular basis by qualified personnel. Instructors should make sure that the equipment is appropriate for the skill level of the class.

- Instructors should arrive before the class starts to check if everything is in working order. They should also look over the equipment and try it out before the class starts.

- They should conduct a weekly inspection of all exercise equipment to ensure that it is operating properly.

- Instructors must regularly check equipment reports to see if any equipment is defective, and then remove or clearly mark any defective equipment to prevent its use.

- They should make sure that they have a good sound system (CD player, volume control, speakers and microphone), and then familiarise themselves with it.

- The classroom floor must absorb the shock from the impact of the participants' movement. A hardwood sprung floor is ideal (Francis 2007). Participants must have enough space to move freely. They should be able to extend their arms to the side and take two steps in any direction without touching another person.

- If possible, all classroom walls should have mirrors in order to allow the participants to see their movements and their posture at all times so they can make corrections if necessary.

- If the class is very large, instructors can lead from a raised platform in order to allow participants in the back row to see them.

- Participants should have easy access to a place to drink water.

- Classrooms should have good ventilation. The temperature should be between 16 and 21 degrees Celsius.

- Instructors must be sure that adequate first aid is available in the facility.

- Instructors must be familiar with medical emergency protocols. They must know how to proceed at any time and in any situation.

Responding Appropriately to a Medical Emergency

The American Heart Association (AHA) and the American College of Sports Medicine (ACSM) recommend that participants in fitness facilities be screened for heart disease with a specially designed questionnaire and that the facility's staff be trained in managing cardiovascular emergencies. Good procedures for preventing cardiovascular events include conducting preparticipation screening, excluding high-risk patients from some activities, reporting and evaluating early symptoms, preparing fitness personnel and facilities for cardiovascular emergencies and recommending prudent exercise programmes (Thompson et al. 2007).

All employees in a fitness centre who directly supervise exercise programmes should be trained in basic life support. Health and fitness facilities must develop and write an appropriate emergency response plan and train their staff in procedures to follow during a life-threatening emergency. In addition, personnel should be familiar with emergency transport teams in the area and should be prepared to help those teams access and locate the centre. Staff should greet the emergency response team at the entrance of the facility so that they can be promptly guided to the site of the emergency. A staff member should remain with the victim at all times (Balady et al. 1998).

The ACSM's guidelines for exercise testing and prescription (2009) describe the key points for a medical emergency plan:

- All staff involved in exercise testing and supervision should be trained in basic cardiopulmonary resuscitation (CPR) and preferably in advanced cardiac life support (ACLS).

- All staff should be trained in how to appropriately handle blood and bodily fluids, and they should be familiar with the risk of blood-borne pathogens according to the OSHA Guidelines for Healthcare Workers (EU-OSHA in Europe).

- One or two trained ACLS personnel and a physician should be immediately available when maximal sign- or symptom-limited exercise testing is being performed.

- All telephones should be clearly labelled with numbers for emergency assistance.

- Written medical emergency plans approved by the medical director should be easily accessible to all staff members.

- Emergency plans should be tested in a specific manner by the facility staff.

- Figures 11.1 and 11.2 describe examples of basic plans for medical incidents with non-emergency situations and for life-threatening situations (ACSM 2009).

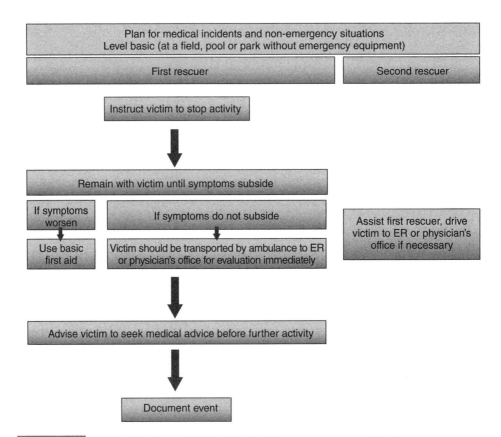

Figure 11.1 Basic plan for medical incidents with non-emergency situations.

Adapted, by permission, from American College of Sports Medicine, 2010, *ACSM's guidelines for exercise testing and prescription,* 8th ed. (Philadelphia (PA): Lippincott Williams & Wilkins), 296.

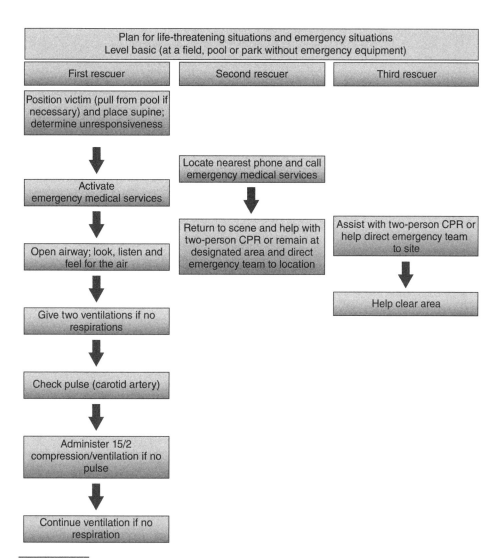

Figure 11.2 Basic plan for life-threatening situations or emergency situations.

Adapted, by permission, from American College of Sports Medicine, 2010, *ACSM's guidelines for exercise testing and prescription,* 8th ed. (Philadelphia (PA): Lippincott Williams & Wilkins), 299.

Conclusion

In order to create an effective group exercise class design, it's necessary to know how to help participants achieve individual objectives, increase physical fitness and improve psychosocial skills. The instructor must stay up to date with new fitness industry techniques and incorporate this information into their class in order for participants to feel welcome and get the most out of their time. It is important that instructors emphasize the importance of fitness gains for the present and the future. After understanding the points presented in this chapter, instructors will be ready to conduct a safe and effective fitness class while avoiding unnecessary risks.

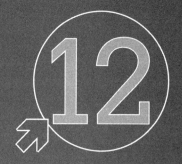

Stress Management Techniques

João Moutão

Susana Franco

This chapter defines the terms *stress*, *distress* and *eustress*, explains the implications of stress and distress on health and well-being, identifies the symptoms of anxiety and depression that may necessitate referral to a medical or mental health professional and provides several relaxation techniques that can be used for stress management.

Stress and Distress

In daily life, the term *stress* is often used to describe negative situations. This leads many people to believe that all stress is bad, which is not true. Actually, some stress is desirable for psychological well-being. *Eustress* (healthy stress) adds excitement, stimulation and colour to life. In contrast, too much stress (*distress*) feels unpleasant, causes anxiety or concern and decreases performance, and it can lead to mental and physical problems (Berger et al 2006). Of course people differ from one another in the optimal levels of stress that are conducive to their personal sense of psychological well-being. Recognising optimal levels of stress and regulating them are important for quality of life.

Another important distinction to make is between acute or short-term stress and chronic stress. The first term refers to a time-limited stress that can occur during a specific situation (e.g., final exams, a blinding snowstorm or a traffic jam). On the other hand, prolonged stress can occur for an indeterminate time period. This type of stress can arise from continuous exposure to a harmful or threatening situation, and it is typically associated with lifestyle, like stressful roles at work or family problems (Lazarus 1999).

Both stress and eustress are individual reactions to events (stressors) that demand change or a response. These desirable or undesirable stressors could originate either in an objective, external context (e.g., starting a new job, getting fired, getting married or becoming a parent) or in the subjective, internal individual perception (e.g., thoughts, interpretations of life events or imagined images). Major undesirable life events are one type of stressor that naturally requires readjustment to the situation. In contrast with major life events, *hassles* are minor sporadic stressors that occur in our everyday lives (e.g., getting a flat tire or misplacing car keys) that can range from irritants to low-intensity stressors, problems and pressures. On the opposite side are pleasurable, uplifting events that make people feel good, like receiving personal compliments, playing sports with friends and watching a good movie. From a mental health viewpoint, it is important that uplifting events occur more often than hassles throughout the day. People can actively cope with stress by striving to overcome its source or by trying to avoid it. They can also cope passively by accepting stress without resistance. In the short term, inappropriate stress management can affect health and well-being.

Implications of Distress for Health and Well-Being

Many people cope with stress by eating, drinking or smoking too much. Others don't deal with it at all. It is now well established that experiencing one or more major negative life events during a 6- to 12-month period has negative implications on health and well-being. When stress reaches a point where it becomes too much (distress), it starts to inhibit mental, emotional and physiological homeostasis. In this condition, the immune system releases the hormone cortisol, also known as the stress hormone. Too much cortisol can make a person susceptible to infection by overly suppressing the immune system, and it can lead to bone loss, muscle atrophy and elevated insulin levels (Buckworth and Dishman 2013).

Too much stress can also affect emotional state, leading to a clinical condition of anxiety and depression. Behaviours that promote wellness include being physically active, choosing a healthy diet, maintaining a healthy body weight, managing stress effectively, avoiding tobacco, limiting alcohol use and protecting against disease and injury (Fahey et al. 2010).

Symptoms of Anxiety and Depression That May Require Professional Attention

According to Knaus (2012) anxiety and depression can have a negative effect on a person's thoughts, feelings and behaviours. Symptoms may include sadness or unhappiness, irritability or frustration, even over small matters, loss of interest or pleasure in normal activities and changes in appetite. Depression can either cause weight loss and decreased appetite, or cause weight gain and increased food cravings. Other symptoms include constant worry and obsession with worst-case scenarios. At the behavioural level, depressed people may cry for no apparent reason, lose their temper easily, feel unsociable, drink and smoke more, experience significant muscle tension or have difficulty sleeping. Some people have symptoms so severe that it's obvious to them that something isn't right. They feel generally miserable or unhappy without really knowing why. In this situation seeing a medical or mental health professional is very important.

Relaxation Techniques

Several relaxation techniques exist for stress management (Anshel 2005; Berger et al. 2006; Gill and Williams 2008), which can be enjoyed in a spa (e.g., sauna, massage), performed in classes (e.g., body and mind, yoga, Pilates) or experienced individually with a specialist. Relaxation techniques that benefit from the mind–body connection can either focus on the body and let the mind follow, or vice versa.

Care in the Application of Relaxation Techniques

Although it is not mandatory to do so, relaxation techniques are usually performed with eyes closed to avoid distractions that come from visual stimulation. If clients are not comfortable doing this, they may leave their eyes open, but health practitioners should encourage clients to close their eyes. Unless the technique requires it, relaxation should be performed without movement.

Relaxation techniques can be performed either while sitting or lying down (supine position), which is a more relaxing position. In the supine position the lower limbs should be placed slightly apart from each other and the upper limbs should be held slightly apart from the trunk, with palms facing upward. A seated position keeps the mind alert, thus preventing sleep, but it may become less comfortable because it requires a greater effort to maintain correct posture in this position. Regardless of the chosen position, the person relaxing must feel comfortable and maintain correct posture.

Preferably, relaxation techniques should be done in a calm and comfortable environment that avoids external disturbances. The room should have low light and an agreeable temperature (not too hot or too cold). Techniques can be performed in silence or to quiet music. Participants should wear comfortable clothing and sit or lie on a comfortable mat.

Breathing

In breathing techniques, participants should inhale through the nose, where the air is warmed, filtered and moistened. Breathing this way also helps keep the sense of smell alive. Participants may exhale through either the nose or the mouth.

Deep breathing is a simple relaxation technique that uses breath to control stress level. Breathing for relaxation should be deep, complete and slow. Participants should inhale through the nose, feeling the air expand the belly first, then the chest (lateral thoracic breathing). Next, they should exhale, releasing air first from the chest and then the belly. Both the inhale and exhale phases must be prolonged. The two phases of breathing can last the same amount of time, or the exhale phase can last longer than the inhale phase, since exhalation has a more relaxing effect of the two. Participants should learn that they can consciously control their breathing.

Another simple technique is breath observation. During this technique, participants simply observe (feel) their breathing as it occurs, without trying to change it. Participants should focus on their breathing, paying attention to the movement of the air during the inhale phase, beginning in the nose and moving into and expanding the trunk. In the exhale phase, they should pay attention to the movement of the air out of the body again as the belly contracts. Breath observation is simultaneously a concentration and a relaxation technique.

Progressive Muscle Relaxation

In 1929 Edmund Jacobson developed the technique of progressive muscle relaxation, which was later adapted by Bernstein and Borkovec in 1973. This technique consists of using progressive contraction and relaxation of muscles in different parts of the body to help people recognise and control their level of muscular tension and relaxation. Initially participants concentrate on the tension induced by voluntarily contracting the muscles, usually for about 5 seconds, and then relaxing that same part of the body. After releasing the muscle, participants should not feel any tension in that area. They can enjoy the feeling of relaxation for 5 to 30 seconds, depending on the available time.

Also, depending on the available time, participants can simultaneously tense and relax more or fewer parts of the body. Ideally participants can go through the body as a whole. If they have more time available, they can apply the technique to the following body segments in this order: right foot, right calf, right thigh, left foot, left calf, left thigh, pelvic area, abdomen, chest, shoulders, back, right hand, right forearm, right upper arm, left hand, left forearm, left upper arm, neck and face. After going through each part of the body, at the end, participants can contract the entire body at once and then relax completely. The technique can be applied to the face as a whole or using smaller parts: forehead, eyes, nose, lips, cheeks, tongue, jaw and chin. If less time is available, participants can use the technique for bigger body segments, such as right lower limb, left lower limb, trunk, right upper limb, left upper limb and face.

Instructors can give prompts for the progressive muscular relaxation technique as follows: 'Contract the right foot and feel the tension', 'Relax the right foot and feel the pleasant sensation of the relaxation, without tension', 'Contract the right leg and focus on the tension', or 'Relax the right leg and feel that part of the body relax, more and more deeply . . .' This technique usually begins with the feet and ends with the head.

Autogenic Training

Autogenic training is a relaxation technique that Johannes Shultz developed in 1930. It consists of self-relaxation of different body areas through continuous concentration and visualisation of sensations (e.g., warmth, cold and heaviness). The technique also focuses on heart rate and breathing. Autogenic training includes the following six stages:

- **Stage 1.** Muscular relaxation experienced by imagining a heavy sensation in different parts of the body (right arm, left arm, both arms, right leg, left leg, both legs, both arms and legs): 'My right arm is heavy; I'm relaxed', 'My left arm is heavy.'

- **Stage 2.** Vascular relaxation experienced by imagining a warm sensation in different body segments (same as stage 1): 'My right arm is warm.'

- **Stage 3.** Cardiac regulation: 'My heartbeat is regular, strong and calm.'
- **Stage 4.** Breathing regulation: 'My breathing is regular, calm and relaxed.'
- **Stage 5.** Regulation of abdominal organs by imagining a warm sensation in the solar plexus (hands can be placed on upper abdominal area): 'My solar plexus is warm.'
- **Stage 6.** Reduction of blood flow to the head: 'My forehead is cool.'

Internal Thoughts and Visualisation

Because thoughts affect feelings, cultivating mental toughness can help control the emotional state. Internal thoughts also affect the level of muscular tension: Positive thoughts reduce the level of muscular tension and negative thoughts increase it (Payne 2005).

For a more positive emotional state, people must realise when negative thoughts appear, stop them and start thinking positively (e.g., trying to be optimistic, seeing the good in the situation, imagining pleasant situations, imagining that they can achieve their goals, trying to believe in themselves and feeling that they are capable).

Mental visualisation can be used as a relaxation technique. Visualisation is a combination of mental representations of reality and imagination. It can focus on cognitive development (e.g., goals, strategies), motor development (e.g., regulation of patterns of an action and sensations that accompany them) or emotional development (e.g., stress management). Mental visualisation can involve all the senses: sight, touch, smell, hearing and taste. Several different things can be visualised: a colour, an energy, a pleasant landscape or scenario, a relaxing situation, a situation in which a goal is reached or other nice things. Visualisation of colours or of energy can be combined with breathing techniques (e.g., 'Imagine you are inhaling energy through your nose, and that energy spreads through your body during exhalation', 'Inhale, breathing in orange light. Feel your energy increasing', or 'Inhale, breathing in blue light that spreads to the most tense zone of your body and helps it relax.').

Meditation

Meditation can be performed for different reasons: to find peace, to raise self-awareness or for illumination. Meditation technique aims to calm the mind and slow thinking. The focus of attention in meditation can include concentrating on breathing (e.g., count the breaths continuously) or on a static image (e.g., sun, moon or a candle) between the eyebrows. During meditation, participants should maintain the focus without analysing it (i.e., they should try not to actively think), allowing their unconscious to express itself. It is natural that after some time, participants may lose focus and start thinking. As soon as they become aware that they have become distracted, they should release their thoughts and return to concentrating on the chosen image or process. Meditation can be performed for anywhere from 5 to 30 minutes, or for even less time (e.g., just 1 minute). Participants just learning to meditate should start by trying this technique for a short duration, and then increasing the time gradually. Because meditation is a very calming technique, participants should perform it in a seated position to avoid falling asleep.

Conclusion

There are different factors that influence people's emotional states, leading to different types of stress (distress and eustress). Both stress and eustress are individual reactions to events (stressors) that demand change or a response and could lead to acute or chronic mental and physical problems. Distress has health and well-being implications, leading to states of anxiety and depression, which may require professional attention. Several relaxation techniques can be used for stress management, such as breathing techniques (e.g., deep breath and breath observation), progressive muscle relaxation, autogenic training, controlled thoughts, visualisation and meditation.

Appendix

European Qualifications Framework (EQF) Level 3: Fitness and Group Fitness Instructor

What Does Level 3 Mean at EQF?

Level of the EQF	Knowledge is described as theoretical or factual.	Skills are described as cognitive (involving the use of logical, intuitive and creative thinking) and practical (involving manual dexterity and the use of methods, materials, tools and instruments).	Competences are described in terms of responsibility and autonomy.
The learning outcomes relevant to level 3	Knowledge of facts, principles, processes and general concepts in a field of work or study.	A range of cognitive and practical skills required for accomplishing tasks and solving problems by selecting and applying basic methods, tools, materials and information.	Take responsibility for completion of tasks in work or study. Adapt own behaviour to circumstances in solving problems.

What Does Level 3 Mean at Fitness QF?

EQF level	Occupation	EuropeActive standards	Target audience
Level 3	**Instructor**[1] **Fitness instructor** Individual instructing **Group fitness instructor** Group instructing: Exercise to music Aquatic exercise Pre-designed programs Other modes of exercise	**EuropeActive level 3** Core fitness Knowledge **EuropeActive level 3 fitness instructor:** Individual fitness additional requirements **EuropeActive level 3 group fitness instructor:** • Music additional requirements • Aquatic additional requirements • Pre-designed additional requirements • Other modes of exercise	General population

[1] It is assumed that the instructor (level 3 EQF) will have acquired all knowledge required to work as a fitness assistant as identified in the *EuropeActive Fitness Assistant Guide* (level 2 EQF, fitness assistant). Thus, these standards should be read in conjunction with *EuropeActive's Foundations for Exercise Professionals,* published by Human Kinetics.

EQF Level 3

Occupational Title

- Fitness instructor
- Group fitness instructor

Purpose of the Job

The purpose of a fitness or group fitness instructor is to build participation of new and existing members through fitness experiences that meet their needs.

Occupational Description

An instructor delivers fitness instruction to individuals with the use of equipment (fitness instructor) or to a group through fitness classes (group fitness instructor). Both types have the same purpose and require the same level of knowledge, skills and competences. Therefore, most of the requirements are the same for both occupations. However, to be able to fulfil this purpose, each of the occupation types may require additional knowledge, skills and competences specific for that type.

Occupational Roles

The fitness or group fitness instructor should be able to do the following:

1. Provide effective and safe fitness instruction
2. Promote healthy lifestyle management
3. Identify individual motives resulting in short-, medium- and long-term fitness goals
4. Suggest relevant exercise adaptations or options to allow for individual client differences or needs
5. Provide participants with advice on intensity and progressing their individual performance and results
6. Observe clients or members at all times and correct unsafe technique
7. Display perfect technique at all times (posture, range of motion, control, timing and form)
8. Positively interact and motivate clients and members using appropriate strategies in order to promote adherence to exercise
9. Deliver good customer service and be a positive role model at all times
10. Promote healthy activities and related strategies for daily living to clients and members (lifestyle management)
11. Promote customer referral: Invite customers to bring friends and family along and promote fitness activities in their social environment
12. Promote a healthy and clean environment
13. Work within the parameters given at level 3, recognizing the standards and professional limitations that this provides and referring to appropriate members of staff for guidance and support

EuropeActive Level 3 Instructor Knowledge Areas

Section 1: Core Fitness Knowledge

Section Overview

- Knowledge and understanding of the principles of human movement and exercise physiology and their application to the components of fitness
- Knowledge of applying the principles of training to each health-related component of fitness

Content Summary and Learning Outcomes

1.1 Human movement

1.1.1 Bones and joints

Instructors should demonstrate knowledge and understanding of the following:

- The major bones and joints and the types of bones and joints
- The structure and function of the skeleton
- The structure and function of the spine and identify normal movement possible at the three main curves

1.1.2 Muscles and muscle actions

Instructors should demonstrate knowledge and understanding of the following:

- The major muscle groups of the body
- The joints crossed by muscle groups
- The principles of paired muscle actions
- The voluntary, involuntary and cardiac muscles
- The basic structure of muscles (muscle fibres, actin and myosin), their role in muscle contraction, connective tissue
- The muscle fibre types (red, white, slow, fast, intermediate, fast, oxidative and glycolytic) and their functions
- The recruitment of fibres in muscle contraction (all-or-none theory)

- The principles of muscle contraction: muscles' cross-joints, muscles only pull, contraction along the line of fibres and working in pairs
- The basic muscle contraction (i.e., concentric, eccentric and isometric (static), prime mover, antagonist and fixator) and the joint actions brought about by specific muscle group contractions

1.1.3 Heart, lungs and circulation

Instructors should demonstrate knowledge and understanding of the following:

- The passage of oxygen through nose, mouth, windpipe and air sacs
- How oxygen and carbon dioxide change places and how oxygen travels to the muscles via the blood
- The action of the diaphragm and the basic mechanics of breathing
- The basic structure of the heart and how blood is pumped and collected
- The link between the heart, lungs and muscles
- The structure and function of arteries, veins, capillaries and mitochondria
- Blood pressure and the effects of exercise
- Short- and long-term effects of exercise on the heart, lungs and circulatory system

1.1.4 Energy systems

Instructors should demonstrate knowledge and understanding of the following:

- The need for energy for muscular contraction
- The role of adenosine diphosphate, adenosine triphosphate (ATP) and creatine phosphate (CP) in energy production for muscular contraction
- Immediate energy: ATP-CP system; short-term energy: the lactic acid system; and long-term energy: the aerobic system
- The aerobic and anaerobic pathways to reform ATP (lactic acid and oxygen)
- The waste products of various forms of physical activity
- The operation of the energy systems in physical activity

- Oxygen debt, oxygen deficit, steady state and $\dot{V}O_2$max
- Food fuels used to provide various types of energy
- The role of intensity and time and individual fitness levels in determining which energy system is used predominantly during exercise
- The muscle fibre types used in relation to aerobic and anaerobic work

1.2 Exercise physiology

1.2.1 Components of fitness

Instructors should demonstrate knowledge and understanding of the following:

- Components of physical fitness
- Components of health-related fitness
- Factors that affect physical fitness
- The relationship between physical fitness, health-related exercise, sport-specific exercise and health

1.2.2 Principles of training

Instructors should demonstrate knowledge and understanding of the following:

- The principles of training
- How the principles of training apply to each of the health-related components of fitness

1.2.3 Muscular strength and endurance

Instructors should demonstrate knowledge and understanding of the following:

- The muscular strength and endurance (MSE) continuum
- The benefits of MSE training in relation to health-related fitness and factors affecting individuals' ability to achieve gains in MSE
- The physiological changes that occur as a result of MSE training
- The principle of overload in FITTA (frequency, intensity, time, type, adherence) applied to muscular strength
- Application of other principles of training to muscular strength and muscular endurance
- The need for the whole-body approach in health-related fitness
- Other activities that will achieve MSE training effect

1.2.4 Aerobic theory

Instructors should demonstrate knowledge and understanding of the following:

- The aerobic–anaerobic continuum
- The physiological and health-related changes that occur as a result of aerobic training
- The benefits of aerobic training
- The differences between and benefits from continuous and interval aerobic training
- Characteristics of aerobic and anaerobic activities: running, walking, sprinting and jumping
- The principle of overload in FITTA (frequency, intensity, time, type, adherence) applied to aerobic training
- Application of all other principles of training to aerobic strength
- Methods of intensity monitoring: heart rate monitoring, rating of perceived exertion and talk test
- Factors affecting an individual's ability to achieve an aerobic training effect
- Structure of the aerobic component in a health-related exercise session: re-warm, peak and cool-down

1.2.5 Stretch theory

Instructors should demonstrate knowledge and understanding of the following:

- Range of movement continuum
- Physiological and health-related changes that occur as a result of stretching
- Types of stretching (dynamic and static)
- Methods of stretching (active and passive)
- Stretch reflex, desensitization and lengthening of muscle tissue (muscle creep)
- Principle of overload in FITTA (frequency, intensity, time, type, adherence) applied to stretching
- Application of all other principles of training to flexibility
- Need for a whole-body approach
- Factors affecting an individual's potential range of movement
- Activities that improve range of movement

1.2.6 Body composition

Instructors should demonstrate knowledge and understanding of the following:

- Basic composition of the human body
- Factors affecting body composition
- The types of basic body composition measurement

1.2.7 Monitoring exercise intensity

Instructors should demonstrate knowledge and understanding of the following:

- Ways of monitoring exercise intensity (taking pulse, rating of perceived exertion, or RPE) and advantages and disadvantages of both
- Personal maximum heart rate estimation and training zones
- The four heart rate training zones
- How the heart rate training zones relate to ratings of perceived exertion and heart rate monitoring

1.2.8 Warm-up

Instructors should demonstrate knowledge and understanding of the following:

- The reasons for warming up
- The physiological changes
- Activities that can be used in a warm-up
- Possible structures of a warm-up
- The importance of specific warm-ups in relation to the chosen type of activity: cardiorespiratory or MSE
- The progress of a warm-up

1.2.9 Cool-down

Instructors should demonstrate knowledge and understanding of the following:

- The reasons for cooling down
- Activities that promote stretching, relaxation and waking up
- Possible structures of a cool-down
- The physiological changes
- Specific cool-downs in relation to the chosen type of activity: cardiorespiratory or MSE

1.2.10 Progression

Instructors should demonstrate knowledge and understanding of the following:

- Relevant physiological changes that occur as a result of changes made to progress a programme over time
- Progressive changes that can be made in terms of overload: frequency, intensity, time, type, adherence, rate, resistance, repetitions, rest and range of movement

1.3 Lifestyle management

1.3.1 Promoting physical activity for health

Instructors should demonstrate knowledge and understanding of the following:

- The cardiorespiratory, muscular and flexibility benefits of physical activity and their relation to reducing risk of disease
- Appropriate exercise activity required for health and fitness (2008 EU Physical Activity Guidelines): health = 30 minutes per day (cumulative) 5 times per week; moderate-intensity fitness = 20 minutes per day (non-stop) 3 times per week; vigorous intensity
- The barriers and motivators to exercise participation
- The exercise prescription for health, well-being and physical fitness
- The agencies involved in promoting physical activity for health in their country
- How to promote a healthy lifestyle: nutrition, opportunities for physical activity in daily life and discourage smoking

1.3.2 Basic nutrition and hydration guidelines

Instructors should demonstrate knowledge and understanding of the following:

- Dietary sources of major nutrients (carbohydrate, fat, protein, vitamins, minerals and fibre)
- Knowledge of the role of carbohydrate, fat and protein as fuels for aerobic and anaerobic metabolism
- The numbers of kilocalories in one gram of carbohydrate, fat, protein and alcohol
- The principle of the balance of energy input (energy intake) and energy output (energy expenditure)

- The definitions of the following terms: obesity, overweight, percentage of body fat, lean body mass and body fat distribution
- The health implications of variation in body fat distribution patterns and the significance of the waist-to-hip ratio, especially the waist perimeter
- The relationship between body composition and health
- The effects of diet plus exercise compared to diet alone and exercise alone as methods for modifying body composition
- The importance of an adequate daily energy intake for healthy weight management
- The myths and consequences associated with inappropriate weight loss methods: saunas, sweat suits and quick-fix diets
- The importance of maintaining proper hydration before, during and after exercise
- The basics of the food pyramid according to the EU, national and local official information

1.3.4 Basic stress management techniques

Instructors should demonstrate knowledge and understanding of the following:

- The definitions of *eustress* and *distress*
- The implications of distress on health and wellbeing
- Possible relaxation techniques: sauna, massage, autogenic training, deep breathing, meditation, progressive muscular relaxation and yoga
- The symptoms of anxiety and depression that may necessitate referral to a medical or mental health professional

1.3.5 Introduction to adaptations and progressions

Instructors should demonstrate knowledge and understanding of the following:

- The facilitator role of the professional regarding the adaptation process in each individual, especially at the beginning of the training process
- The importance of providing a proper dose–response relationship according to the level of the individual
- The importance of a good communication strategy regarding the training adaptation process

1.4 Health and safety

1.4.1 Safe and effective exercise

Instructors should demonstrate knowledge and understanding of the following:

- Individual fitness levels, posture, range of motion, body type, movement control, intensity, temperature, form, timing, skeletal alignment, previous injury and exercise history
- Movements for safety and effectiveness applying the previously listed conditions
- Ways of reducing the risks associated with unsafe exercise

1.4.2 Modifications to exercise: alternatives and adjustments

Instructors should demonstrate knowledge and understanding of the following:

- Individual and group performance needs and exploring appropriate exercise options or alternatives according to fitness level and health status

1.4.3 Body awareness and exercise technique

Instructors should demonstrate knowledge and understanding of the following:

- The importance of being a role model in exercise performance and technique
- How to correct posture and body alignment, range of motion, control, timing and form for all fitness exercises
- The control of static and dynamic movement and spatial awareness

1.4.4 Health and safety, dealing with accidents and emergencies

Instructors should demonstrate knowledge and understanding of the following:

- The national legal responsibilities of fitness or group fitness instructors
- National and local requirements and procedures in the working environment, risk assessment and identifying procedures
- Methods of dealing with emergencies according to internationally recognized procedures (e.g., *AHA/ACSM Joint Statement:*

Recommendations for Cardiovascular Screening, Staffing, and Emergency Policies at Health and Fitness Facilities, 1998)

1.4.5 Legal requirements and emergency procedures

Instructors should demonstrate knowledge and understanding of the following:

- Legal responsibilities and accountability when dealing with the public and awareness of the need for honesty and accuracy in substantiating claims of authenticity when promoting services in the public domain
- A responsible attitude about the care and safety of participants in the training environment and in planned activities ensuring that both are appropriate to the needs of the clients
- Ensuring appropriate liability and indemnity insurance to protect clients
- An absolute duty of care in awareness of working environment and ability to deal with all reasonably foreseeable accidents and emergencies—and to protect themselves, colleagues and clients

1.4.6 Professionalism, code of practice, ethics, national standards and guidelines

Instructors should demonstrate knowledge and understanding of the following:

- The EuropeActive and EREPS code of ethical practice included (see www.ereps.eu for more information)

1.5 Communication

1.5.1 Building rapport

Instructors should demonstrate knowledge and understanding of the following:

- How to connect with people
- How to learn and remember people's names
- Effective use of voice and body language
- Empathetic listening (listening to understand instead of listening to reply)
- Praising and encouraging positive behaviour
- Showing genuine interest in the individual
- Use of open-ended questions reflecting answering

1.5.2 Motivational strategies

Instructors should demonstrate knowledge and understanding of the following:

- Learning individual reasons or motives behind people's exercise goals
- The most important and effective behavioural strategies for enhancing exercise and health behaviour change (e.g. reinforcement, goal setting, social support, problem solving, reinforcement strategies and self-monitoring)
- Stages of change of the transtheoretical model and the ability to use basic strategies for various stages
- Definitions and practical examples of extrinsic and intrinsic reinforcement

1.5.3 Customer service

Instructors should demonstrate knowledge and understanding of the following:

- Definition of the exercise customer
- Welcoming and receiving the customer
- Service-oriented concepts
- Approaching and responding to customers in a positive way
- Principles of customer service
- Avoiding and dealing with conflict
- Being open and friendly all the time
- Methods and practices that contribute to effective customer care
- Skills of effective customer care: communication, body language and negotiation

Section 2: Description of the Fitness Instructor Occupation

A fitness instructor welcomes, introduces and adheres members to fitness by providing inductions to new members and ongoing programmes to existing members. These inductions and following programmes need to be planned, instructed and evaluated. A fitness instructor coaches members through these programmes and is responsible for the resulting experience, which should be positive and meet the member's wants and needs. The role includes actively promoting and encouraging joining and adhering to regular exercise.

Additional specific roles

- Collect and check information relating to individual clients
- Analyse information relating to individual clients
- Plan, instruct and evaluate safe and appropriate gym-based exercise sessions
- Provide one-to-one or group inductions and general exercise programmes, including the introduction to new equipment where appropriate
- Select relevant exercises and design appropriate programmes that address safety at all times
- Use logical and progressive teaching methodologies to introduce a range of exercises in relation to clients' goals
- Select and correctly demonstrate a variety of cardiorespiratory and resistance training methods that can be used by clients or members
- Provide clients or members with general advice on progressing individual programmes

Additional specific requirements: section overview

In addition to the core fitness knowledge, a fitness instructor must master the following additional knowledge, skills and competences:

- Ability to design, instruct and evaluate individual fitness programs and sessions
- Basic understanding of health and safety issues, including responding to emergencies
- Basic understanding of the skills involved in supporting participants in developing and maintaining fitness

Content Summary and Learning Outcomes

2.1 Individual instruction—core knowledge

2.1.1 Designing an individual fitness programme

Instructors should demonstrate knowledge and understanding of the following:

- The structure of an individual fitness programme: warm-up, main activity and cool-down

- The design of an individual fitness programme
- The necessary skills of an effective and qualified fitness instructor

2.1.2 Delivering a fitness session

Instructors should demonstrate knowledge and understanding of the following:

- The national legal responsibilities of the fitness instructor
- Identifying status of participants relative to screening information
- Identifying any changes required (alternatives or adaptations) to planned activities
- Health and safety checks relevant to the exercise environment
- The information needed for responding appropriately to a medical emergency
- Providing an appropriate plan for the sessions

2.1.3 Information gathering, screening and informed consent

Instructors should demonstrate knowledge and understanding of the following:

- Importance of gathering information before the start of the session in relation to the participants and their needs
- Reasons for screening, advantages and disadvantages of verbal and written screening, purpose of the PAR-Q and informed consent as a health and safety requirement, participant expectations and motivation, extent of previous exercise participation and current level of ability
- The EuropeActive Health Fitness Code of Ethics or national standards and guidelines with reference to competence, confidentiality, safety—this is specific to each country, or adopt EuropeActive's code of ethics

2.1.4 Ending a session, evaluating and giving and receiving feedback

Instructors should demonstrate knowledge and understanding of the following:

- Giving feedback to participants regarding their performance
- Gathering information from participants to improve personal performance
- Identifying other sources of feedback: managers, coordinators and colleagues

- Using appropriate questions to gain relevant information
- Evaluating own performance against criteria on observation checklist
- Ensuring participants leave the fitness environment safely
- Putting equipment away and assessing for future use
- Leaving environment in safe condition for future use
- Informing or agreeing with participants on time, location and content of further sessions

2.1.5 Planning of safe progressive exercise

Instructors should demonstrate knowledge and understanding of the following:

- The relevance of physiological changes occurring in the body and how to progress exercises over time
- The progressive changes that can be made in terms of overload: frequency, intensity, time, type and adherence; principles of training such as specificity, progressive overload and reversibility

2.2 Resistance exercise

2.2.1 Resistance machine lifts (including warm-up)

Instructors should demonstrate knowledge and understanding of the following:

- Terms and definitions in resistance training
- Correct lifting technique for all exercises on resistance machines: leg press, leg extension, leg curl, seated and standing calf raise, bench press, pec dec, pullover, shoulder press, lateral raise, upright row, seated row, lat pully, bicep curl, triceps pushdown, hip extension, seated abduction and seated adduction
- Correct machine setup and adjustment and variables appropriate to each machine (e.g., seat height, point of pivot and lever length)
- The primary and secondary (where relevant) muscle groups involved in each exercise
- Which exercises are multi-joint and which are single-joint exercises and their suitability for beginners
- Warming up specifically for resistance training
- Pros and cons of the use of cardiovascular (CV) machines or body weight for warming up

2.2.2 Free weights (standing)

Instructors should demonstrate knowledge and understanding of the following:

- Correct lifting technique for standing free weight (barbells or dumbbells) lifts: deadlift, upright row, front raise, bicep curl, lateral raise, squat, lunge, shoulder press and triceps extension
- Correct body alignment and weight distribution through every phase of each exercise
- Primary and secondary (where relevant) muscle groups involved in each exercise
- Which exercises are multi-joint and which are single-joint exercises and their suitability for beginners
- Various adaptations that may be required to allow for individual differences

2.2.3 Free weights (seated) including spotting

Instructors should demonstrate knowledge and understanding of the following:

- Correct lifting technique for free-weight lifts using a bench: bench press (flat/incline), lying triceps extension, single-arm row, bent-arm pullover, supine dumbbell fly (flat/incline), dumbbell chest press, dumbbell prone fly or prone row
- Safe and effective spotting techniques
- Various adaptations that may be required to allow for individual differences

2.2.4 Practical guidelines for instructing resistance training

Instructors should demonstrate knowledge and understanding of the following:

- How to demonstrate and practice resistance exercises by naming the exercise, naming the general area of the body, naming the target muscle (primary mover), performing a silent demonstration of the exercise, explaining the demonstration, instructing customer into the correct position by giving the key points (including individual questioning and feedback) and individually correcting and adjusting

2.2.5 Methods of resistance training

Instructors should demonstrate knowledge and understanding of the following:

- A variety of resistance training methods and systems (e.g., pyramid, circuit and superset)
- The value of using these accordingly in relation to the individual's goals
- The dose–response relationship of these methods based on actual evidence

2.3 Cardiorespiratory exercise

2.3.1 Cardiorespiratory machines

Instructors should demonstrate knowledge and understanding of the following:

- Correct technique for using CV machines: treadmill, rower, stepper, upright bike, recumbent bike, elliptical trainer and cross-trainer
- Correct setup of machines, variables appropriate to each machine and individual adjustment (e.g., seat height, duration and speed)

2.3.2 Methods of cardiovascular training

Instructors should demonstrate knowledge and understanding of the following:

- A variety of cardiorespiratory training methods and discussing their value according to participant needs (e.g., continuous or interval)
- The dose–response relationship based on actual evidence

Section 3: Description of the Group Fitness Instructor Occupation

A group fitness instructor welcomes, introduces and adheres members to fitness by providing group classes to new and existing customers. These classes need to be delivered effectively and safely. A group fitness instructor coaches customers through these classes and is responsible for their fitness experience, which should be positive and meet the customers' wants and needs. The role also includes actively promoting and encouraging joining and adhering to regular exercise.

Additional specific roles

- Explain the benefits of the particular group fitness programme.
- Demonstrate and explain exercises to a group and correct incorrect technique of individual participants.

- Create a positive, encouraging social atmosphere and group interaction.
- Interact with participants before and after class.

Additional specific requirements

In addition to the core fitness knowledge, a group fitness instructor must master the following additional knowledge, skills and competences:

- The ability to plan, teach and evaluate group fitness classes
- Basic understanding of health and safety issues, including responding to emergencies
- Basic understanding and application of the skills involved in supporting participants in developing and maintaining fitness

Content Summary and Learning Outcomes

3.1 Group fitness instruction—core knowledge

3.1.1 Gather participant information

Instructors should demonstrate knowledge and understanding of the following:

- The importance of gathering information before the start of the class in relation to the participants and their needs: new participants, programme experience, names, inquiring about injuries, checking correct gear, the EuropeActive Health Fitness Code of Ethics or national standards and guidelines with reference to competence, confidentiality, safety specific to each country or adopting EuropeActive's code of ethics

3.1.2 Inform participants of programme benefits and target audience

Instructors should demonstrate knowledge and understanding of the following:

- Programme exercise goals and benefits and required level of fitness to participate
- For whom the programme is suitable and not suitable
- Intensity and impact options

3.1.3 Delivering a group fitness class

Instructors should demonstrate knowledge and understanding of the following:

- How to design or deliver content in a pre-designed group fitness programme
- For whom the programme is suitable and not suitable
- Intensity and impact options
- National legal responsibilities of a group fitness instructor
- Identifying any changes required (options, alternatives or adaptations) to planned exercises
- The information needed to respond appropriately to a medical emergency

3.1.4 Ending a class and giving and receiving feedback

Instructors should demonstrate knowledge and understanding of the following:

- Giving feedback to the group and individual participants regarding their performance
- Using appropriate questions to gain relevant information
- Evaluating own performance against programme guidelines and criteria
- Ensuring participants leave the class safely
- Leaving environment in safe condition for future use
- Thanking and inviting participants to the next class

3.2 Group fitness to music

3.2.1 Teaching group fitness to music

Instructors should demonstrate knowledge and understanding of the following:

- How to move to the beat of the music
- The structure of a group fitness class to music: warm-up, main activity and cool-down
- The required skills of an effective instructor of group fitness to music
- How to use music to motivate participants
- The basic moves for a self-designed group fitness class to music
- The exact moves in a pre-designed exercise class to music
- How to move in all movement planes and use directional changes
- How to make transitions and link exercises

- How to verbally and visually cue and instruct exercise routines timely and clearly, including the use of body language, voice projection, teaching points and demonstrations from different angles and visual previews

3.2.2 Music and choreography

Instructors should demonstrate knowledge and understanding of the following:

- The advantages and disadvantages of using music
- The slow and fast beat (i.e., beats per minute)
- The upbeat and the downbeat
- Appropriate music and beats for various components of a class
- Using music phrasing for exercise movement
- National legal requirements and responsibilities relating to the use of music
- The ways music can be used: background or choreographed
- How music is built up: verse, pre-chorus, chorus, instrumental and bridges

3.2.3 Methods of choreography

Instructors should demonstrate knowledge and understanding of the following:

- How to design choreography using various methods (including layering and holding patterns) and learn pre-designed choreography according to specific programme guidelines
- How to correctly deliver self- or pre-designed programme specific choreography

3.2.4 Guidelines for group fitness to music

Instructors should demonstrate knowledge and understanding of the following:

- Legal and insurance responsibilities in respect of the national guidelines
- Identifying any changes required (alternatives or adaptations) to planned class activity, identifying health and safety checks relevant to the exercise environment and identifying the information needed for responding appropriately to a medical emergency

References

Chapter 1

Afthinos Y., N.D. Theodorakis, P. Nassis. 2005. Customers' expectations of service in Greek fitness centers: Gender, age, type of sport center, and motivation differences. *Managing Service Quality* 15 (3): 245–258.

Alexandris K., P. Zahariadis, C. Tsorbatzoudis, G. Grouios. 2004. An empirical investigation of the relationships among service quality, customer satisfaction and psychological commitment in a health club context. *European Sport Management Quarterly* 4 (1): 36–52.

Anderson E.W., C. Fornell, D.R. Lehmann. 1994. Customer satisfaction, market share, and profitability: Findings from Sweden. *Journal of Marketing* 58 (3): 53–66.

Bitner, M.J. 1992. Servicescapes: The impact of physical surroundings on customers and employees. *Journal of Marketing* 56 (2): 57–71.

Bodet, G. 2008. Customer satisfaction and loyalty in service: Two concepts, four constructs, several relationships. *Journal of Retailing and Consumer Services* 15 (3): 156–162.

Brehm W., J. Eberhardt. 1995. Drop-out und Bindung im Fitness-Studio. *Sportwissenschaft* 25 (2): 174–186.

Eckmann. 2007. Focusing on customer service. In: Bates M., editor. *Health fitness management: A comprehensive resource for managing and operating programs and facilities.* 2nd ed. Champaign (IL): Human Kinetics. p. 171-184.

German Fitness Gym Association. 2013. *Eckdaten der deutschen Fitnesswirtschaft 2012.* Hamburg (Germany): SSV-Verlag.

Grönroos, C., editor. 2007. *Service management and marketing: Customer management in service competition.* Chichester (UK): Wiley.

Hallowell, R. 1996. The relationship of customer satisfaction, customer loyalty, and profitability: An empirical study. *International Journal of Service Industry Management* 7 (4): 27–42.

Homburg C., N. Koschate. 2007. Kundenzufriedenheit und Kundenbindung. In: S. Albers, A. Herrmann, editors. *Handbuch Produktmanagement.* 3rd ed. Wiesbaden (Germany): Gabler. p. 843-867.

Howat G., J. Absher, G. Crilley, I. Milne. 1996. Measuring customer service quality in sports and leisure centres. *Managing Leisures* 1 (2): 77–89.

Ko Y.J., D.L. Pastore. 2004. Current issues and conceptualizations of service quality in the recreation sport industry. *Sport Marketing Quarterly* 13: 159–167.

Lagrosen S., Y. Lagrosen. 2007. Exploring service quality in the health and fitness industry. *Managing Service Quality* 17 (1): 41–53.

Lengnick-Hall, C.A. 1996. Customer contribution to quality: A different view of the customer-oriented firm. *Academy of Management Review* 21 (3): 791–824.

Meffert H., M. Bruhn, editors. 2008. *Dienstleistungsmarketing: Grundlagen – Konzepte –Methoden.* 6th ed. Wiesbaden (Germany): Gabler.

Moxham C., F. Wiseman. 2009. Examining the development, delivery and measurement of service quality in the fitness industry: A case study. *Total Quality Management & Business Excellence* 20 (5): 467–482.

Rampf, J. 1999. *Drop-Out und Bindung im Fitness-Sport. Günstige und ungünstige Bedingungen für Aktivitäten im Fitness-Studio.* Hamburg (Germany): Czwalina.

Rieger, T. 2009. Erfolgreiche Kunden sind treue Kunden. *Fitness Tribune* 21 (4): 18, 149.

Rieger, T. 2011. Erfolgsfaktor Mitarbeiterorientierung—Zur Bedeutung des Internen Marketing für kommerzielle Fitnesssportanbieter. *Sciamus—Sport und Management* 2 (2): 40–50.

Scharnbacher K., G. Kiefer. 2003. *Kundenzufriedenheit: Analyse, Messbarkeit und Zertifizierung.* 3rd ed. Munich (Germany): Oldenbourg.

Schneider B., D. Bowen. 1995. *Winning the service game.* Boston (MA): Harvard Business School Press.

Stauss B., W. Seidel. 2007. *Beschwerdemanagement: Unzufriedene Kunden als profitable Zielgruppe.* 4th ed. Munich (Germany): Carl Hanser.

Tsitskari E., D. Tsiotras, G. Tsiotras. 2006. Measuring service quality in sport services. *Total Quality Management & Business Excellence* 17 (5): 623–631.

Zeithaml V.A., M.O. Bitner, D.D. Gremler, editors. 2012. *Services marketing.* 6th ed. New York (NY): McGraw-Hill.

Zollner, G. 1995. *Kundennähe in Dienstleistungsunternehmen. Empirische Analyse von Banken.* Wiesbaden (Germany): Gabler.

Chapter 2

Abraham A., D. Collins. 2006. The coaching schematic: Validation through expert coaches consensus. *Journal of Sport Sciences* 24 (6): 549–564.

Benda R. 2006. Sobre a natureza da aprendizagem motora: Mudança e estabilidade... e mudança. *Revista Brasileira Educação Física e Esporte* 20: 43–45. Available from: www.gedam.com.br/publi/artigos/Benda_2006.pdf.

Bodet G. 2006. Investigating customer satisfaction in a health club context by an application of the Tetraclasse Model. *European Sport Management Quarterly* 6: 149–165.

Castañer M., O. Camerino, M.T. Anguera, G.K. Jonsson. 2010. Observing the paraverbal communicative style of expert and novice PE teachers by means of SOCOP: A sequential analysis. *Procedia—Social and Behavioral Sciences* 2 (2): 5162–5167.

Chin K. 2005. The effects of the teacher's feedback during badminton instruction. In: F. Carreiro da Costa, M. Cloes, M. Valeiro, editors. *The art and science of teaching in physical education and sport.* Lisbon (Portugal): FMH. Serviço de Edições. p. 139-147.

Côté J., W. Sedgwick. 2003. Effective behaviors of expert rowing coaches: A qualitative investigation of Canadian athletes and coaches. *International Sports Journal* 7 (1): 62–77.

Fernandéz J., G. Carrión, D. Ruíz. 2012. La satisfacción de clientes y su relación con la percepción de calidad en Centros de Fitness: Utilización de la escala CALIDFIT. *Revista de Psicología del Deporte* 21 (2): 309–319. Available from: http://ddd.uab.cat/pub/revpsidep/revpsidep_a2012v21n2/revpsidep_a2012v21n2p309.pdf.

Franco F. 2002. El tratamiento de la información. La necessidad del feedback. *Revista Digital* Año 8 (50). Available from: www.efdeportes.com.

Franco S., V. Simões. 2006. *Participants' perception and preference about Body Pump® instructors' pedagogical feedback.* Paper presented at the 11th annual Congress of the European College of Sport Science, Lausanne, Switzerland.

Gusthart J., I. Kelly, J. Rink. 1997. The validity of the qualitative measures of teaching performance scale as a measure of teacher effectiveness. *Journal of Teaching in Physical Education* 16: 196–210.

Kennedy C., M. Yoke. 2005. *Methods of group exercise instruction.* Champaign (IL): Human Kinetics.

Knop P.D. 2004. Quality management in sports clubs. *Sport Management Review* 7 (1): 57–77.

Molinero O., A. Salguero, B. Tabernero, C. Tuero, S. Márquez. 2005. El abandono deportivo: Propuesta para la intervención práctica en edades tempranas. *Revista Digital* Año 10 (90). Available from: www.efdeportes.com.

Murcia J., L. Oliveira. 2002. Diferenças motivacionais na aprendizagem e desenvolvimento de programas de natação e de fitness aquático. *Fitness & Performance Journal* 1 (2): 42–51.

Papadimitriou A., K. Karteroliotis. 2000. The service quality expectations in private sport and fitness centers: A reexamination of the factor structure. *Sport Marketing Quarterly* 9 (3): 157–164.

Pedragosa V., A. Correia. 2009. Expectations, satisfaction and loyalty in health and fitness clubs. *International Journal of Sport Management and Marketing* 5 (4): 450–463.

Piéron M. 1996. *Formação de professores. Aquisição de técnicas de ensino e supervisão pedagógica.* Cruz Quebrada (Portugal): Serviço de Edições da Faculdade de Motricidade Humana.

Piéron M. 1999. *Para una enseñanza eficaz de las actividades físico-deportivas.* Barcelona (Spain): INDE Publicaciones.

Rinne M., E. Toropainen. 1998. How to lead a group—Practical principles and experiences of conducting a promotional group in health-related physical activity. *Patient Education and Counseling* 33: 69–76.

Rosado A., L. Virtuoso, I. Mesquita. 2004. Relação entre as competências de diagnóstico de erros das habilidades técnicas e a prescrição pedagógica no voleibol. *Revista Brasileira de Educação Física e Esporte* 18 (2): 151–157.

Sarmento P. 2004. *Pedagogia do desporto e observação.* Cruz Quebrada (Portugal): Edições Faculdade de Motricidade Humana.

Seibert R., L. Francis. 2000. Group fitness instructor manual. ACE's guide for fitness professionals. In: D. Green, editor. *Teaching a group exercise class.* San Diego (CA): ACE. p. 179-204.

Silva I.L., H. Beresford. 2004. A percepção da linguagem não-verbal ou corporal como meio de se interpretar o moral ou estado de animo de atletas submetidos a um treinamento de alto nível de performance. *Fitness & Performance Journal* 3 (6): 351–357.

Simões V., R. Santos-Rocha. 2015/*In Press.* Body awareness and exercise technique. In: F. Naclerio, T. Rieger, A. Jiménez, editors. *EuropeActive's foundations for exercise professionals.* Champaign (IL): Human Kinetics.

Woo B., P. Chelladurai. 2012. Dynamics of perceived support and work attitudes: The case of fitness club employees. *Human Resource Management Research* 2 (1): 6–18.

Young D., A. King. 2000. Group fitness instructor manual. ACE's guide for fitness professionals. In: D. Green, editor. *Adherence and motivation.* San Diego (CA): ACE. p. 206-225.

Chapter 3

Chung M.K., M.W. Rich. 1990. Introduction to the cardiovascular system. *Alcohol Health and Research World* 14 (4): 269–276.

Fox S.M., J.P. Naughton, W.L. Haskell. 1971. Physical activity and the prevention of coronary heart disease. *Annals of Clinical Research* 3: 404–432.

Garber C.E., B. Blissmer, M.R. Deschenes, B.A. Franklin, M.J. Lamonte, I.M. Lee, D.C. Nieman, D.P. Swain. 2011. American College of Sports Medicine position stand. Quantity and quality of exercise for developing and maintaining cardiorespiratory, musculoskeletal, and neuromotor fitness in apparently healthy adults: Guidance for prescribing exercise. *Medicine & Science in Sports & Exercise* 43 (7): 1334–1359.

Gellish R.L., B.R. Goslin, R.E. Olson, A. McDonald, G.D. Russi, V.K. Moudgil. 2007. Longitudinal modelling of the relationship between age and maximal heart rate. *Medicine & Science in Sports & Exercise* 39 (5): 822–829.

Giese M. 1988. Organization of an exercise session. In: American College of Sports Medicine, editor. *Resource manual for guidelines for exercise testing and prescription.* Philadelphia (PA): Lippincott Williams and Wilkins. p. 244-247.

Institute of Medicine of the National Academies of Science. 2002. *Dietary reference intakes for energy, carbohydrate, fibre, fat, fatty acids, cholesterol, protein, and amino acids (macronutrients).* Washington (DC): National Academy Press.

McArdle W., V.L. Katch. 1996. *Exercise physiology: Energy, nutrition, and human performance.* Philadelphia (PA): Lippincott Williams and Wilkins.

Physical Activity Guidelines Advisory Committee. 2008. *Physical Activity Guidelines Advisory Committee report.* Washington (DC): U.S. Department of Health and Human Services.

Tanaka H., K.D. Monahan, D.R. Seals. 2001. Age-predicted maximal heart rate revisited. *Journal of the American College of Cardiology* 37: 153–156.

Chapter 4

American College of Sports Medicine (ACSM). 2002. Progression models in resistance training for healthy adults, American College Of Sport Medicine, position stand. *Medicine & Science in Sports & Exercise* 34: 364–380.

American Heart Association and American College of Sports Medicine (AHA/ACSM). 1998. Scientific statement recommendations for cardiovascular screening, staffing, and emergency policies at health/fitness facilities. *Circulation* 97: 2283–2293.

Andersen J.C. 2005. Stretching before and after exercise: Effect on muscle soreness and injury risk. *Journal of Athletic Training* 40: 218–220.

Bishop D. 2003a. Warm-up I. Potential mechanisms and the effects of passive warm-up on exercise performance. *Sports Medicine* 33: 439–454.

Bishop D. 2003b. Warm-up II. Performance changes following active warm-up and how to structure the warm-up. *Sports Medicine* 33: 483–498.

Buchanan C.I., R.L. Marsh. 2002. Effects of exercise on the biomechanical, biochemical and structural properties of tendons. *Comp Biochem Physiol A Mol Integr Physiol* 133: 1101–1107.

Colado J.C., X. Garcia-Masso. 2009. Technique and safety aspects of resistance exercises: A systematic review of literature. *The Physician and Sportsmedicine* 37: 104–111.

Donnelly D.V., W.P. Berg, D.M.T. Fiske. 2006. The effect of the direction of gaze on the kinematics of the squat exercise. *Journal of Strength and Conditioning Research* 20: 145–150.

Durall C.J., R.C. Manske, G.J. Davies. 2001. Avoiding shoulder injury from resistance training. *Strength and Conditioning Journal* 23: 10–18.

Earle R.W., T.R. Baechle. 2008. Strength training and spotting techniques. In: T.R. Baechle and R.W. Earle, editors. *Essentials of strength training and conditioning.* 3rd ed. Champaign (IL): Human Kinetics.

Escamilla R.F. 2001. Knee biomechanics of the dynamic squat exercise. *Medicine & Science in Sports & Exercise* 33: 127–141.

Faigenbaum, A.D., G.D. Myer. 2012. Exercise deficit disorder (EDD) in youth: Play now or pay later. *Current Sports Medicine Reports* 11 (4): 196–200.

Faigenbaum A.D., G. Myer, F. Naclerio, A. Casas. 2011. Injury trends and prevention in youth resistance training. *Strength and Conditioning Journal* 33 (3): 36–41.

Faigenbaum A.D., N.S. Liatsos. 1994. The use and abuse of weightlifting belts. *Strength and Conditioning Journal* 16 (4): 60–62.

Greenwood, M., L. Greenwood. 2008. Facility organization and risk management. In: T.R. Baechle and R.W. Earle, editors. *Essentials of strength training and conditioning.* 3rd ed. Champaign (IL): Human Kinetics.

Halson S.L., A.E. Jeukendrup. 2004. Does overtraining exist? An analysis of overreaching and overtraining research. *Sports Medicine* 34 (14): 967–981.

Harman E. 1994. Weight training safety: A biomechanical perspective. *Strength and Conditioning Journal* 16 (5): 55–60.

Harman E. 2008. Biomechanics of resistance exercise. In: T.R. Baechle and R.W. Earle, editors. *Essentials of strength training and conditioning.* 3rd ed. Champaign (IL): Human Kinetics.

Heiderscheit B.C., M.A. Sherry, A. Silder, E.S. Chumanov, D.G. Thelen. 2010. Hamstring strain and injuries: Recommendation for diagnosis, rehabilitation, and injury prevention. *Journal of Orthopaedic & Sports Physical Therapy* 40 (2): 67–81.

Jeffreys I. 2008. Warm-up and stretching. In: T.R. Baechle and R.W. Earle, editors. *Essentials of strength training and conditioning.* 3rd ed. Champaign (IL): Human Kinetics.

Jones C.S., C. Christensen, M. Young. 2000. Weight training injury trends: A 20-year survey. *The Physician and Sportsmedicine* 28 (7): 61–72.

Kay A.D., A.J. Blazevich. 2012. Effect of acute static stretch on maximal muscle performance: A systematic review. *Medicine & Science in Sports & Exercise* 44 (1): 154–164.

Kellis E., F. Arambatzi, C. Papadopoulos. 2005. Effects of load reaction force and lower limb kinematics during concentric squat. *Journal of Sports Sciences* 23 (10): 1045–1055.

Klein K.K. 1961. The deep squat exercise as utilized in weight training for athletes and its effect on the ligaments of the knee. *J. Assoc. Phys. Ment. Rehabil.* 15: 6–11.

Krieger J.W. 2009. Single versus multiple sets of resistance exercise: A meta-regression. *Journal of Strength and Conditioning Research* 23 (6): 1890–1901.

Krieger J.W. 2010. Single versus multiple sets of resistance exercise for muscle hypertrophy: A meta-analysis. *Journal of Strength and Conditioning Research* 24 (4): 1150–1159.

Lander J.E., J.R. Hundley, R.L. Simonton. 1992. The effectiveness of weight belts during multiple repetitions of the squat exercise. *Medicine & Science in Sports & Exercise* 24 (5): 603–609.

Li G., E. Most, L.E. Defrate, J.F. Suggs, T.J. Gill, H.E. Rubash. 2004. Effect of the posterior cruciate ligament on posterior stability of the knee in high flexion. *Journal of Biomechanics* 37 (5): 779–783.

McHugh M.P., C.H. Cosgrave. 2010. To stretch or not to stretch: The role of stretching in injury prevention and performance. *Scandinavian Journal of Medicine & Science in Sports* 20 (2): 169–181.

Myer G.D., C.E. Quatman, J. Khoury, E.J. Wall, T.E. Hewett. 2009. Youth versus adult "weightlifting" injuries presenting to United States emergency rooms: Accidental versus nonaccidental injury mechanisms. *Journal of Strength and Conditioning Research* 23 (7): 2054–2060.

Naclerio F. 2009. Valoración de la fuerza en el entrenamiento personal. In: G. Hernando, editor. *Nuevas tendencias en el entrenamiento personal.* Barcelona (Spain): Paidotribo.

Naclerio F., D. Forte. 2011. Entrenamiento de fuerza y su relación con la prevención de lesiones en el deporte. In: F. Naclerio, editor. *Entrenamiento deportivo, fundamentos y aplicaciones en diferentes deportes.* Madrid (Spain): Médica Panamericana.

Naclerio F., M. Rhea, P. Marín. 2011. Entrenamiento de fuerza para mejorar el rendimiento deportivo. In: F. Naclerio, editor. *Entrenamiento deportivo, fundamentos y aplicaciones en diferentes deportes.* Madrid (Spain): Médica Panamericana.

Neitzel J.A., G.J. Davies. 2000. The benefits and controversy of the parallel squat in strength training and rehabilitation. *Strength and Conditioning Journal* 22 (3): 30–37.

Olsen L., A. Scanian, M. Mackay, S. Babul, D. Reid, M. Clark, P. Raina. 2004. Strategies for prevention of soccer related injuries: A systematic review. *British Journal of Sports Medicine* 38 (1): 89–94.

Olsen O.E., G. Myklebust, L. Engebretsen, I. Holme, R. Bahr. 2005. Exercises to prevent lower limb injuries in youth sports: Cluster randomised controlled trial. *British Medical Journal* 330 (7489): 449.

Pappas A.M., T.P. Goss, P.K. Kleinman. 1983. Symptomatic shoulder instability due to lesions of the glenoid labrum. *American Journal of Sports Medicine* 11 (5): 279–288.

Peterson M.D., M.R. Rhea, B.A. Alvar. 2005. Application of the dose-response for muscular strength: A review of meta-analytic efficacy and reliability for designing training prescription. *Strength and Conditioning Journal* 19 (4): 950–958.

Ratamess N. 2012a. Resistance training equipment and safety. In: N. Ratamess, editor. *ACSM's foundations of strength training and conditioning.* Philadelphia (PA): Lippincott Williams and Wilkins.

Ratamess N. 2012b. Warm-up and flexibility. In: N. Ratamess, editor. *ACSM's foundations of strength training and conditioning.* Philadelphia (PA): Lippincott Williams and Wilkins.

Ratamess N. 2012c. Resistance training program design. In: N. Ratamess, editor. *ACSM's foundations of strength training and conditioning.* Philadelphia (PA): Lippincott Williams and Wilkins.

Renfro G.J., W.P. Ebben. 2006. A review of the use of lifting belts. *Strength and Conditioning Journal* 28 (1): 68–74.

Schoenfeld B.J. 2010. Squatting kinematics and kinetics and their application to exercise performance. *Journal of Strength and Conditioning Research* 24 (12): 3497–3506.

Shoemaker S.C., K.L. Markolf. 1985. Effects of joint load on the stiffness and laxity of ligament-deficient knees. *The Journal of Bone & Joint Surgery* 67 (1): 136–146.

Siff M.C. 2004. *Supertraining.* Denver (CO): Supertraining Institute.

Stone M., H.S. O'Bryant, C. Ayers, W.A. Sands. 2006. Stretching: Acute and chronic? The potential consequences. *Strength and Conditioning Journal* 28 (6): 66–74.

Thacker S.B., J. Gilchrist, D.F. Stroup, C.D. Kimsey, Jr. 2004. The impact of stretching on sports injury risk: A systematic review of the literature. *Medicine & Science in Sports & Exercise* 36 (3): 371–378.

Tillin N.A., D. Bishop. 2009. Factors modulating post-activation potentiation and its effect on performance of subsequent explosive activities. *Sport Medicine* 39 (2): 147–166.

Yack H.J., C.E. Collins, T.J. Whieldon. 1993. Comparison of closed and open kinetic chain exercise in the anterior cruciate ligament-deficient knee. *The American Journal of Sports Medicine* 21 (1): 49–53.

Young W.B. 2007. The use of static stretching in warm-up for training and competition. *International Journal of Sports Physiology and Performance* 2 (2): 212–216.

Zatsiorsky V.M., J.W. Kraemer. 2006. *Sciences and practice of strength training.* Champaign (IL): Human Kinetics.

Chapter 5

American College of Sports Medicine (ACSM). 2009. *ACSM's guidelines for exercise testing and prescription.* 8th ed. Philadelphia (PA): Lippincott Williams & Wilkins.

Anderson K., D.G. Behm. 2005. The impact of instability resistance training on balance and stability. *Sports Medicine* 35 (1): 43–53.

Baechle T.R., R.W. Earle, editors. 2008. *Essentials of strength training and conditioning.* 3rd ed. Champaign (IL): Human Kinetics.

Earle R.W., T.R. Baechle, editors. 2004. *Essentials of personal training.* Champaign (IL): Human Kinetics.

Fitzgerald G.K., J.D. Childs, T.M. Ridge, J.J. Irrgang. 2002. Agility and perturbation training for a physically active individual with knee osteoarthritis. *Physical Therapy* 82 (4): 372–382.

Fleck S.J., W.J. Kraemer. 2004. *Designing resistance training programs.* Champaign (IL): Human Kinetics.

Garber C.E., B. Blissmer, M.R. Deschenes, et al. 2011. American College of Sports Medicine position stand. Quantity and quality of exercise for developing and maintaining cardiorespiratory, musculoskeletal, and neuromotor fitness in apparently healthy adults: Guidance for prescribing exercise. *Medicine & Science in Sports & Exercise* 43 (7): 1334–1359.

Hass C.J., M.S. Feigenbaum, B.A. Franklin. 2001. Prescription of resistance training for healthy populations. *Sports Medicine* 31 (14): 953–964.

Howley E.T., D.L. Thompson. 2012. *Fitness professional's handbook.* 6th ed. Champaign (IL): Human Kinetics.

Issurin V.B. 2010. New horizons for the methodology and physiology of training periodization. *Sports Medicine* 40 (3): 189–206.

Kraemer W.J., K. Adams, E. Cafarelli, et al. 2002. American College of Sports Medicine position stand. Progression models in resistance training for healthy adults. *Medicine & Science in Sports & Exercise* 34 (2): 364–380.

Murphy M.H., S.N. Blair, E.M. Murtagh. 2009. Accumulated versus continuous exercise for health benefit: A review of empirical studies. *Sports Medicine* 39 (1): 29–43.

Peterson M.D., M.R. Rhea, B.A. Alvar. 2005. Applications of the dose-response for muscular strength development: A review of meta-analytic efficacy and reliability for designing training prescription. *Journal of Strength & Conditioning Research* 19 (4): 950–958.

Phillip S.M. 2009. Physiologic and molecular bases of muscle hypertrophy and atrophy: Impact of resistance exercise on human skeletal muscle (protein and exercise dose effects). *Applied physiology, nutrition, and metabolism* 34 (3): 403–410.

Rhea M.R., B.A. Alvar, L.N. Burkett, S.D. Ball. 2003. A meta-analysis to determine the dose response for strength development. *Medicine & Science in Sports & Exercise* 35 (3): 456–464.

Swain D.P., B.A. Franklin. 2006. Comparison of cardioprotective benefits of vigorous versus moderate intensity aerobic exercise. *American Journal of Cardiology* 97 (1): 141–147.

Swain D.P., B.C. Leutholtz. 2007. *Exercise prescription: A case study approach to the ACSM guidelines.* 2nd ed. Champaign (IL): Human Kinetics.

Wilmore J.H., D.L. Costill, W.L. Kenney. 2008. *Physiology of sport and exercise,* 4th ed. Champaign (IL): Human Kinetics.

Chapter 6

American College of Sports Medicine (ACSM). 2009. *ACSM's guidelines for exercise testing and prescription.* 8th ed. Philadelphia (PA): Lippincott Williams & Wilkins.

American College of Sports Medicine (ACSM). 2011. Quantity and quality of exercise for developing and maintaining cardiorespiratory, musculoskeletal, and neuromotor fitness in apparently healthy adults: Guidance for prescribing exercise. American College of Sport Medicine: Position stand. *Medicine & Science in Sports & Exercise* 43 (7): 1334–1359.

Canadian Society for Exercise Physiology. 2002. *The Physical Activity Readiness Medical Examination* (PARmed-X). Available from: http://www.csep.ca/cmfiles/publications/parq.pdf Corbin C.B., R. Lindsey. 1994. *Concepts in physical education with laboratories.* 8th ed. Dubuque (IA): Times Mirror Higher Education Group.

Canadian Society for Exercise Physiology. 2013. *The Physical Activity Readiness Medical Examination for Pregnancy* (PARmed-X for PREGNANCY). Available from: http://www.csep.ca/cmfiles/publications/parq/parmed-xpreg.pdf

Doran G.T. 1981. There's a S.M.A.R.T. way to write management's goals and objectives. *Management Review* 70 (11): 35–36.

Gormley S.E., D.P. Swain, R. High, R.J. Spina, E.A. Dowling, U.S. Kotipalli, R. Gandrakota. 2008. Effect of intensity of aerobic training on $\dot{V}O_2$max. *Medicine & Science in Sports & Exercise* 40 (7): 1336–1343.

Griffin J.C. 1998. *Client-centered exercise prescription.* Champaign (IL): Human Kinetics.

Hardman A.E., D. Stensel. 2003. *Physical activity and health. The evidence explained.* London (UK): Routledge.

Heyward V. 2010. *Advanced fitness assessment and exercise prescription.* Champaign (IL): Human Kinetics.

Pedersen B.K., B. Saltin. 2006. Evidence for prescribing exercise as therapy in chronic disease. *Scandinavian Journal of Medicine & Science in Sports* 16 (suppl. 1): 3–63.

Physical Activity Guidelines Advisory Committee. 2008. *Physical Activity Guidelines Advisory Committee Report.* Washington (DC): U.S. Department of Health and Human Services.

Swain D.P., B.A. Franklin. 2006. Comparison of cardioprotective benefits of vigorous versus moderate intensity aerobic exercise. *The American Journal of Cardiology* 97 (1): 141–147.

U.S. Department of Health and Human Services.1996. *Physical activity and health: A report of the Surgeon General.* Atlanta (GA): U.S. Department of Health and Human Services, Centers for Disease Control and Prevention, National Center for Chronic Disease Prevention and Health Promotion.

U.S. Department of Health and Human Services. 2008. *Physical activity guidelines for Americans.* Available from: www.health.gov/paguidelines.

Wilmore J.H., D.L. Costill. 1994. *Physiology of sport and exercise.* Champaign (IL): Human Kinetics.

Chapter 7

Aerobics and Fitness Association of America (AFFA). 2002. *Fitness theory and practice.* 4th ed. Sherman Oaks (CA): Author.

American College of Sports Medicine (ACSM). 2009. *ACSM's guidelines for exercise testing and prescription.* 8th ed. Philadelphia (PA): Lippincott Williams & Wilkins.

Appel A. 2007. The right rehearsal. *IDEA Fitness Journal* January: 94.

Baechle T.R., R.W. Earle, editors. 2008. *Essentials of strength training and conditioning.* 3rd ed. Champaign (IL): Human Kinetics.

Barth J., S. Schneider, R. von Kanel. 2010. Lack of social support in the etiology and the prognosis of coronary heart disease: A systematic review and meta-analysis. *Psychosomatic Medicine* 72 (3): 229–238.

Clark C.M. 2005. Relations between social support and physical health. *Personality Papers.* Available from: www.personalityresearch.org/papers/clark.html.

Heather M.A. 2006. Depression, isolation, social support, and cardiovascular disease in older adults. *Journal of Cardiovascular Nursing* 21 (5): S2–S7.

Howley E.T., B.D. Franks. 2007. *Fitness professional's handbook.* Champaign (IL): Human Kinetics.

IDEA. 2005. Group fitness instructor code of ethics. *IDEA Fitness Journal* February: 67.

Kennedy C. 2003. Functional exercise progression. *IDEA Personal Trainer* February: 36–43.

Kennedy C.A., M.M. Yoke. 2005. *Methods of group exercise instruction.* Champaign (IL): Human Kinetics.

Kennedy-Armbruster C., M.M. Yoke. 2009. *Methods of group exercise instruction.* 2nd ed. Champaign (IL): Human Kinetics.

Kuper H., H.O. Adami, T. Theorell, E. Weiderpass. 2006. Psychosocial determinants of coronary heart disease in middle-aged women: A prospective study in Sweden. *American Journal of Epidemiology* 164: 349–357.

McGonigal K. 2007. Facilitating fellowship. *IDEA Health and Fitness Journal* June: 73–79.

Nieman D.C. 2003. *Exercise testing and prescription: A health-related approach.* 5th ed. Boston (MA): McGraw-Hill.

Yoke M., C. Kennedy. 2004. *Progressive functional training.* Monterey (CA): Healthy Learning.

Chapter 8

Franco S., R. Santos. 1999. *A essência da ginástica aeróbica.* Rio Maior (Portugal): Edições ESDRM.

Hayakawa Y., H. Miki, K. Takada, K. Tanaka. 2000. Effects of music on mood during bench stepping exercise. *Perceptual and Motor Skills* 90 (1): 307–314.

Karageorghis C.I., Priest D.L. Music in the exercise domain: a review and synthesis (Part I). International review of sport and exercise psychology. 2012 Mar;5(1):44-66.

Karageorghis C.I., P.C. Terry, A.M. Lane, D.T. Bishop, D.L. Priest. 2012. The BASES Expert Statement on use of music in exercise. *Journal of Sports Sciences* 30 (9): 953–956.

Santos-Rocha R., C. Oliveira, A. Veloso. 2006. Osteogenic index of step exercise depending on choreographic movements, session duration and stepping rate. *British Journal of Sports Medicine* 40 (10): 860–866.

Santos-Rocha R., A. Veloso, M.L. Machado. 2009. Analysis of ground reaction forces in step-exercise depending on step-pattern and stepping-rate. *Journal of Strength and Conditioning Research* 23 (1): 209–224.

Turner C.H., A.G. Robling. 2003. Designing exercise regimens to increase bone strength. *Exercise and Sport Sciences Reviews* 31 (1): 45–50.

Chapter 9

Franco S., R. Santos. 1999. *A essência da ginástica aeróbica.* Rio Maior (Portugal): Edições ESDRM.

Hayakawa Y., H. Miki, K. Takada, K. Tanaka. 2000. Effects of music on mood during bench stepping exercise. *Perceptual and Motor Skills* 90 (1): 307–314.

Karageorghis CI, Priest DL. Music in the exercise domain: a review and synthesis (Part I). International review of sport and exercise psychology. 2012 Mar;5(1):44-66.

Santos-Rocha R., C. Oliveira, A. Veloso. 2006. Osteogenic index of step exercise depending on choreographic movements, session duration and stepping rate. *British Journal of Sports Medicine* 40 (10): 860–866.

Santos-Rocha R., A. Veloso, M.L. Machado. 2009. Analysis of ground reaction forces in step-exercise depending on step-pattern and stepping-rate. *Journal of Strength and Conditioning Research* 23 (1): 209–224.

Turner C.H., A.G. Robling. 2003. Designing exercise regimens to increase bone strength. *Exercise and Sport Sciences Reviews* 31 (1): 45–50.

Chapter 10

American College of Sports Medicine (ACSM). 2013. Behavioral theories and strategies for promoting exercise. In: L.S. Pescatello, editor. *ACSM's guidelines for exercise testing and prescription.* 9th ed. Baltimore (MD): Lippincott, Williams and Wilkins. p. 355–382.

Ashford S., J. Edmunds, D.P. French. 2010. What is the best way to change self-efficacy to promote lifestyle and recreational physical activity? A systematic review with meta-analysis. *British Journal of Health Psychology* 15 (Pt 2): 265–288. PubMed PMID: 19586583.

Bandura A. 1977. Self-efficacy: Toward a unifying theory of behavioral change. *Psychological Review* 84 (2): 191–215. PubMed PMID: 847061.

Bonelli S. 2000. *Step training.* Exercise ACo, editor. San Diego (CA): American Council on Exercise. p. 90

Hutchison A.J., J.D. Breckon, L.H. Johnston. 2009. Physical activity behavior change interventions based on the transtheoretical model: A systematic review. *Health Education & Behavior: The official publication of the Society for Public Health Education* 36 (5): 829–845. PubMed PMID: 18607007.

Martin S.B. 2013. Principles of behaviour change: Skill building to promote physical activity. In: A.K. Swain, editor. *ACSM's resource manual for guidelines for exercise testing and prescription.* Baltimore (MD): Lippincott, Williams and Wilkins. p. 745–760.

McClanahan B.S. 2013. Counselling physical activity behavior change. In: A.K. Swain, editor. *ACSM's resource manual for guidelines for exercise testing and prescription.* Baltimore (MD): Lippincott, Williams and Wilkins. p. 761–773.

Napolitano M.A. 2013. Theoretical foundations of physical activity behavior change. In: A.K. Swain, editor. *ACSM's resource manual for guidelines for exercise testing and prescription.* Baltimore (MD): Lippincott, Williams and Wilkins. p. 730–744.

Prochaska J.O., C.C. DiClemente, J.C. Norcross. 1992. In search of how people change. Applications to addictive behaviors. *The American Psychologist* 47 (9): 1102–1114. PubMed PMID: 1329589.

Silva M.N., D. Markland, C.S. Minderico, P.N. Vieira, M.M. Castro, S.R. Coutinho, et al. 2008. A randomized controlled trial to evaluate self-determination theory for exercise adherence and weight control: Rationale and intervention description. *BMC Public Health* 8 (234). PubMed PMID: 18613959. Pubmed Central PMCID: 2483280.

Spencer L., T.B. Adams, S. Malone, L. Roy, E. Yost. 2006. Applying the transtheoretical model to exercise: A systematic and comprehensive review of the literature. *Health Promotion Practice* 7 (4): 428–443. PubMed PMID: 16840769.

Teixeira P.J., E.V. Carraca, D. Markland, M.N. Silva, R.M. Ryan. 2012. Exercise, physical activity, and self-determination theory: A systematic review. *Int J Behav Nutr Phys Act.* 9: 78. PubMed PMID: 22726453. Pubmed Central PMCID: 3441783.

Chapter 11

American College of Sports Medicine (ACSM). 2010. *ACSM's guidelines for exercise testing and prescription.* 8th ed. Philadelphia (PA): Lippincott Williams & Wilkins.

Balady G.J., B. Chaitman, D. Driscoll, et al. 1998. Recommendations for cardiovascular screening, staffing and emergency policies at health/fitness facilities. *Circulation* 97: 2283–2293.

Connaughton D.P. 1998. The changing standard of care and the legal implications for recreational sports and fitness facility administrators. *Recreational Sports Journal* 22 (3): 20–22.

Francis, L.L. 2007. Teaching a group exercise class. In: American Council of Exercise, editor. *ACE group fitness instructor manual. A guide for fitness professionals.* 2nd ed. Monterey (CA): Healthy Learning: 200-224.

Herbert D.L. 1996. Legal and professional responsibilities of personal training. The business of personal training. In: S.O. Roberts, editor. *The business of personal training.* Champaign (IL): Human Kinetics: p. 53-63 .

McCann E.H. 1998. Legal aspects of fitness programs and facilities. *Recreational Sports Journal* 12 (2): 20–23.

Thompson P.D., B.A. Franklin, G.J. Balady, et al. 2007. Exercise and acute cardiovascular events: Placing the risk into perspective: A scientific statement from the American Heart Association Council on Nutrition, Physical Activity, and Metabolism and the Council on Clinical Cardiology. *Circulation* 115 (17): 2358–2368.

Chapter 12

Anshel M.H. 2005. Strategies for preventing and managing stress and anxiety in sport. In: D. Hackfort, J. L. Duda, R. Lidor, editors. *Handbook of research in applied sport and exercise psychology: International perspectives.* Morgantown (WV): Fitness Information Technology. p. 199-215.

Berger B., D. Pargman, R. Weinberg. 2006. *Foundations of exercise psychology.* 2nd ed. Morgantown (WV): Fitness Information Technology.

Bernstein D.A., T. D. Borkovec. 1973. *Progressive relaxation training: A manual for the helping professions.* Champaign (IL): Research Press.

Buckworth J., R. Dishman. 2013. *Exercise psychology.* 2nd ed. Champaign (IL): Human Kinetics.

Fahey T.D., P.M. Insel, W.T. Roth. 2013. *Fit & well.* 10th ed. New York (NY): McGraw-Hill.

Gill D.L., L. Williams. 2008. *Psychological dynamics of sport and exercise.* 3rd ed. Champaign (IL): Human Kinetics.

Knaus W.J. 2012. *The cognitive behavioral workbook for depression. A step by step program.* 2nd ed. Oakland (CA): New Harbinger Publications.

Lazarus R. 1999. *Stress and emotion: A new synthesis. London (England): Free Association Books.*

Payne R.A. 2005. *Relaxation techniques: A practical handbook for the health care professional.* 3rd ed. London (England): Elsevier.

Index

Note: The italicized *f* and *t* following page numbers refer to figures and tables, respectively.

About the Editors

Rita Santos Rocha, PhD, is an associate professor at the Sport Sciences School of Rio Maior (ESDRM) Polytechnic Institute of Santarém, Portugal. Since 1998, she has been teaching courses in physical activity and public health, exercise testing and prescription and exercise biomechanics. Dr. Santos Rocha is also a researcher at CIPER (Neuromechanics of Human Movement Group) of the Faculty of Human Kinetics, University of Lisbon. Her research projects are funded by the Portuguese Foundation for Science and Technology and the European Union National Strategic Reference Framework in the fields of active pregnancy, active school, active ageing and biomechanics. She is a member of the scientific committee of the Gymnastics Federation of Portugal and vice chair of the standards council of EuropeActive. Dr. Santos Rocha has a BSc in sport sciences, MSc in exercise and health and PhD in human movement for health and fitness. In the past, she was a fitness instructor, group gymnastics coach, and physical education teacher.

Thomas Rieger is the chairman of the standards council of Europe Active. He holds a doctoral degree in social sciences with a specialization in sport science (German PhD equivalent) from the University of Tübingen and a master's degree in public health. In 2007, he was appointed as a professor of sport management at the Business and Information Technology School (BiTS) in Iserlohn, Germany. At BiTS, he is the vice dean of the bachelor's programme of sport and event management and the MSc programme of international sport and event management. Previously, Dr. Rieger served as the visiting professor at the Real Madrid Graduate School and the European University Cyprus in Nicosia. Before entering academia in 2006, he gained more than six years of experience in the fitness industry, especially in the fields of fitness marketing and quality management.

Alfonso Jiménez is a professor of exercise and health and the faculty dean of the health, exercise and sport sciences department at European University of Madrid (Spain) and a member of the scientific advisory board of UKActive Research Institute. Dr. Jiménez holds a visiting professorial appointment at Victoria University in Melbourne, Australia, as the international research associate. He is the chair of the Fitness Australia/ISEAL research programme and scientific advisory committee at the University of Greenwich in London. During the time that he was head of school and deputy dean at Victoria University, Dr. Jiménez served as a professor and head of the Centre for Sports Sciences and Human Performance at the University of Greenwich. From 2009 to 2012, Professor Jiménez was the chairman of the standards council of EuropeActive, which at the time was called the European Health & Fitness Association. He was awarded honorary membership in recognition of his outstanding service. Dr. Jiménez's background before entering academia centred on the fitness industry in management, research and sales.

Contributors

Paolo Benvenuti
Technogym Research Department, Italy

Oscar Carballo Iglesias
UC, Departamento de Educación Física e Deportiva. *Facultade de Ciencias do Deporte e a Educación Física, Universidade da Coruña* (Department of Physical Education and Sports. Faculty of Sport Sciences and Physical Education – University of A Coruña), A Coruña, Spain

Susana Franco
ESDRM-IPS, *Escola Superior de Desporto de Rio Maior - Instituto Politécnico de Santarém* (Sport Sciences School of Rio Maior - Polytechnic Institute of Santarém), Portugal

Sonia García Merino
UEM, *Facultad de Ciencias de la Actividad Física y el Deporte - Universidad Europea de Madrid* (Faculty of Physical Activity and Sport Sciences - European University of Madrid), Spain

Jana Havrdová
FISAF International, FISAF.cz, Czech Chamber of Fitness, Prague, Czech Republic

Eliseo Iglesias-Soler
UC, Departamento de Educación Física e Deportiva. *Facultade de Ciencias do Deporte e a Educación Física, Universidade da Coruña* (Department of Physical Education and Sports. Faculty of Sport Sciences and Physical Education – University of A Coruña), A Coruña, Spain

Alfonso Jiménez
UEM, *Facultad de Ciencias de la Actividad Física y el Deporte - Universidad Europea de Madrid* (Faculty of Physical Activity and Sport Sciences - European University of Madrid), Spain

Jeremy Moody
UWIC, Cardiff School of Sport, Cardiff Metropolitan University, Cardiff, Wales, United Kingdom

Susana Moral González
UEM, *Facultad de Ciencias de la Actividad Física y el Deporte - Universidad Europea de Madrid* (Faculty of Physical Activity and Sport Sciences - European University of Madrid), Spain

João Moutão
ESDRM-IPS, *Escola Superior de Desporto de Rio Maior - Instituto Politécnico de Santarém* (Sport Sciences School of Rio Maior - Polytechnic Institute of Santarém), Portugal

Fernando Naclerio
Centre of Sport Sciences and Human Performance School of Science, University of Greenwich, Kent, United Kingdom

Simona Pajaujiene
LSU, Lithuanian Sport University, Kaunas, Lithuania

Nuno Pimenta
ESDRM-IPS, *Escola Superior de Desporto de Rio Maior - Instituto Politécnico de Santarém* (Sport Sciences School of Rio Maior - Polytechnic Institute of Santarém), Portugal

Thomas Rieger
BiTS, Business and Information Technology School, Faculty of International Service Industries, Germany

Rita Santos Rocha
ESDRM-IPS, *Escola Superior de Desporto de Rio Maior - Instituto Politécnico de Santarém* (Sport Sciences School of Rio Maior - Polytechnic Institute of Santarém), Portugal

Vera Simões
ESDRM-IPS, *Escola Superior de Desporto de Rio Maior - Instituto Politécnico de Santarém* (Sport Sciences School of Rio Maior - Polytechnic Institute of Santarém), Portugal

Lenka Velínská
FISAF, *Česká komora fitness* (Czech Aerobic, Fitness and Dance Organization), Prague, Czech Republic

Silvano Zanuso
Technogym Research Department, Italy

About EuropeActive

The European Register of Exercise Professionals uses the Europe Active standards as its quality assurance process to ensure that exercise professionals are suitably qualified to offer safe and effective fitness programmes to their clients all across Europe. EREPS provides consumers, employers and partners in medical professions with the necessary level of confidence that registered trainers are competent and work to support its Code of Ethical Practice which defines the rights and principles of being an exercise professional. By referencing the EuropeActive standards to each trainer and by being registered it means that they have met the prescribed minimum standards of good practice, that they are committed to raising their standards, skills and professional status through a process of lifelong learning.

EREPS is regulated by the EuropeActive Standards Council using the accepted official European Qualification Framework which describes the knowledge, skills and competencies exercise professionals need to achieve for registration.

About the EuropeActive Series

Endorsed by EuropeActive, the continent's leading standard-setting organisation in fitness and health, these texts are the authoritative guides for current and future exercise professionals and training providers in Europe.

Authored by renowned experts from all over Europe, the information in these texts ranges from foundational knowledge to specific practical essentials for exercise professionals. For those who promote physical activity and healthier lifestyles, there are no other titles with more authority in Europe.

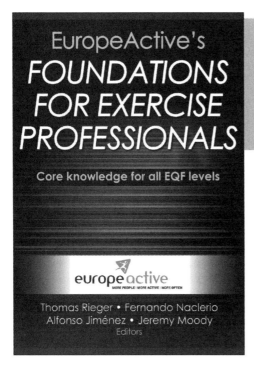

EuropeActive's Foundations for Exercise Professionals
EuropeActive
Thomas Rieger, Fernando Naclerio, Alfonso Jiménez, and Jeremy Moody, Editors
©2015 • Hardback • Approx. 352 pp
Print: ISBN 978-1-4504-2377-9
E-book: ISBN 978-1-4925-0577-8

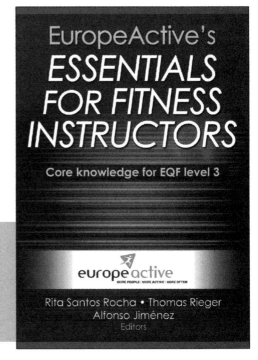

EuropeActive's Essentials for Fitness Instructors
EuropeActive
Rita Santos Rocha, Thomas Rieger, and Alfonso Jiménez, Editors
©2015 • Hardback • Approx. 208 pp
Print: ISBN 978-1-4504-2379-3
E-book: ISBN 978-1-4925-0591-4

Find out more at www.HumanKinetics.com!

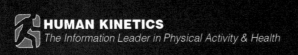

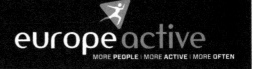